OWN YOUR

ADHD

DISCOVER YOUR TRUE POTENTIAL

FAIGY LIEBERMANN
ADHD SUCCESS COACH &
PROFESSIONAL ORGANISER

The information in this book is complete to the best knowledge of the
author Faigy Liebermann. All recommendations are made without
guarantee on the part of the author. The author disclaims any liability in
connection with the use of this information for personal, business, medical
or public use.

The information in this book is presented to expand your awareness of the
many ways to support your ADHD. The information in this book is meant
to supplement, not replace, proper treatment. Before practicing the skills
described in this book, be sure that you have asked the advice of a
competent mental health professional.

In the client stories all names and identifying details have been changed to
protect the privacy of individuals. Any resemblance to actual persons,
living or dead, or actual events is purely coincidental.

This book is not intended as a substitute for the medical advice of
physicians. The reader should regularly consult a physician in matters
relating to his/her health, and particularly with respect to any symptoms
that may require diagnosis or medical attention.

OWN YOUR

ADHD

DISCOVER YOUR TRUE POTENTIAL

"Whether you think you may have ADHD, are newly diagnosed with ADHD, or you have had your diagnosis for some time, 'Own Your ADHD – Discover Your True Potential' is a must have, effective resource full of up-to-date information, case studies and strategies to help you own your ADHD and take your rightful place in the world."

Andrea Bilbow OBE
Founder of ADDISS and President of ADHD Europe

"A great overview of ADHD and how to manage its accompanying challenges and strengths. Useful for anyone with the condition or trying to understand it on behalf of a family member, loved one or colleague. I personally used one of the tips for managing 'hypofocus' this morning and it worked great! Thank you, Faigy!"

Michelle Beckett
CEO, ADHD Action

"I recommend this book. Faigy provides an easy to read step-by-step journey through the day-to- day impact of living with an ADHD brain whilst providing some simple but highly effective strategies to uncover and build on the strengths of living with ADHD, supporting the reader to find the tools to reach their true potential."

Rob Baskind
Consultant psychiatrist Adult ADHD

"Faigy Lieberman has written a highly readable book that will help make sense of ADHD, providing very practical strategies for dealing with the challenging symptoms of ADHD. Using real examples from her coaching experience, Faigy provides the reader with opportunities to discover their true potential – becoming the victor, not victim of their ADHD."

Tracy Dickens
ADHD Foundation

"In the second of Faigy's wonderful publications she gives an informative yet distinctly human approach to the dilemmas faced by those with ADHD. The book and illustrations take the reader on a rhythmical journey through the mind. You will not only learn about the psychological theories that give fabulous insight about Executive Function, you will also find out how a difference in this area will look, sound and feel through the real client experiences. This book is a brilliant coaching tool for anyone interested in how people think, with clever narrative that allows the reader to understand the ideas in a more personal way, or pick up and go to a specific section that is time relevant to them."

Sarah Musique
Executive performance coach

"ADHD is a tremendous gift when you understand it correctly. Unfortunately, the common scenario is that too many years are wasted until you understand your ADHD correctly. You can try to cope alone do it the long, slow and painful way, or you can read this book; a gift given to you by Faigy Liebermann. In 'Own Your ADHD – Discover Your True Potential', you will develop an in depth understanding of your ADHD and how to work successfully with it. Faigy hands over her vast experience in this field. I recommend that everyone who has the gift of ADHD reads her book."

Aharon Lerner
Author of "Pathways to Success"
Psychotherapist

CONTENTS

PART 1
WELCOME

MY LIFE WITH ADHD

The term ADHD means Attention Deficit Hyperactivity Disorder. It is commonly thought that ADHD refers to difficulty in focusing. The heart of the ADHD challenge is the difficulty regulating one's emotions. Do you recognise yourself or someone you love in my story?

I am married, I am a mum with five children, one of whom has been diagnosed with ADHD together with ASD.

In 2013 I trained as a professional organiser. I quickly noticed similar challenges among my clients. I trained further at ADDCA, the gold standard in ADHD coach training, to learn the skills I needed to help my clients succeed with their ADHD.

I remember the place where I was standing and listening to the lecturer explain what ADHD really is. I felt as if I had been struck by a flash of lightning understanding. So, it's me. I have ADHD. That was a life-changing moment. I see my life as before that moment and afterward.

Over the next few years my understanding of ADHD deepened, especially the understanding of ADHD in women.

I started to think of myself as having an ADHD personality. After all, I am organised, focused and great with my time management. I don't have proper ADHD, right? Wrong!

As my ADHD understanding deepened, I realised that I have high functioning ADHD, and the symptoms in women differ greatly to the ADHD symptoms in men.

Here are my top 3 strengths (typical ADHD):

- High energy, and motivation in my areas of passion
- Vision
- Foresight

I love organising, I do not hoard. It can't be that I have

ADHD... (I have realised that my ADHD brain craves the dopamine hit that I get when I work with my clients to part with an item of clutter, and help them get their homes organised...)

Here are my 3 top weaknesses which are typical ADHD:

- Poor (or non-existent) working memory
- High emotional volatility
- Anxiety

I attributed my very high anxiety levels as a teen and young adult to my difficult childhood.

I had super social phobia up till my 30s...

Now it all makes sense...

GETTING MY ADHD DIAGNOSIS

I only received a formal ADHD diagnosis in November 2019, as a result of talking to an ADHD professional. He advised me that I should get an ADHD assessment as I so clearly showed the classical signs of ADHD in women. I still didn't really believe that I had ADHD. I wanted to understand the ADHD diagnosis experience that my clients go through. So I booked an appointment, (private as that is the only way that you can be seen quickly here in the UK).

When I filled out the forms, I didn't know what was going on! Every single one of those questions applied to me! It was not surprising that during the first session I got diagnosed with ADHD. When the diagnostician asked me if I wanted ADHD meds I agreed right away.

I wanted to go on medication to understand how my clients feel when they are on the meds. I was still convinced that I did not really have ADHD, and the meds wouldn't work right? I was prescribed Concerta. I received got the meds 2 days later. Whether I had ADHD or not I wanted to experience what my clients feel. I know there's a lot of stigma attached to the ADHD meds, and it is mostly from ignorance. ADHD is one of the most commonly studied mental health conditions. Over 100,000 studies have been conducted on ADHD.

The first day I took only 1 tablet, (18mg) with the aim of raising the dose to 2 tablets 7 days later and 3 tablets 14 days later.

You know what they say, if the ADHD meds works then you have ADHD. If they don't work, then you probably don't have ADHD. The first week the meds had no effect whatsoever the only difference was after on the first day around 4pm when the meds wore off I felt decidedly odd for a couple of minutes. I knew I had to be patient. So the second week I was very eager to see if there was a difference when taking 2 tables (36mg)

I was disappointed that there was no difference. Maybe I didn't have ADHD after all...

YES, I HAVE ADHD!!

During week 2 I took 2 tablets for 3 days then I forgot to take the dose for two days. On the 5th day I left the house early for an appointment, I was aware of a distinctly nervous feeling and I was aware that I was driving too fast. I realised I hadn't felt like this in a while. I realised that the meds must be working after all... I must have ADHD...

I got back at 10am and took 2 tablets. Since I hadn't taken them for 2 days, I felt a bit "off." I pushed through. Around 2pm I noticed that I felt calmer.

This was on Friday. I am Jewish and we observe the Sabbath. Sabbath comes in at sundown. In the winter this is really early around 3.30pm.

After I had lit the candles and welcomed the Sabbath. I sat down with my 7-year-old son to play with him. This is our weekly ritual. Every week I tell him that this is the best time of the week for me! I tell him that I just love to play with him and can't wait for this time. I don't tell him that it is the hardest time of the week…This week I sat down and played a game with my 7-year-old son for 45 minutes without getting up once.

I listened to a detailed account from my teenage daughter for 20 minutes…with patience and focus, and it was actually interesting…

Suddenly everything is coming into focus. I feel like my glasses prescription has been fixed! I didn't even know it was faulty… I am not looking out at the world in a fog anymore.

MANAGING IMPULSIVITY AND SELF-CONTROL

The most amazing change is, that food is no longer "talking to me" and "pulling me"

I served a 3-course meal on Friday night. I was full after the second course. I did not touch the third course, my favourite, Chinese chicken, even when I was busy serving and clearing up…for the first time in my life.

My thoughts were focused! No jumble, no tangle. Just one thought at a time.

For the last 3 years I've had a diet coach attend my home for weekly sessions. I am 5 foot 5 inches, and a regular size 14. Since forever, and especially the last 5 years I have felt that something was "off." It was so very hard to eat a balanced diet and have self-control.

Since the meds started working, my level of feeling in control regarding food has turned around 360 degrees.

To be fair I had worked mightily hard to instil good eating habits. Now all the meds do is take away that edge if impulsivity/self- control challenge. I bake for my family on a weekly basis. I usually bake a batch of wholemeal cupcakes and biscuits. With my full-time job .and being a busy mum, I still manage to fit in home baking in my week. (I put into practise the tools I teach my clients…)

Post meds, I am not tempted anymore to take a quick nibble or bite. This is even when the meds where off. Premeds, I would have had a mighty hard daily battle with myself not to eat any.

Whenever I had to play with the kids or listen to long detailed conversations... or do boring tasks, I used to have a physical pain in my brain that has been accompanying me since forever. That feeling is gone.

There was a minor extended family crisis on Friday afternoon. I handled it calmly. Later that evening, I discussed this incident with my daughter and my husband. Listening to myself, I couldn't believe that I was able to keep my voice at a calm level, and calmly explain myself... This had NEVER happened before... No hysterical histrionics, no drama queen... Just clear, calm and solution oriented.

I am currently on 72 mg of Concerta, which is well below the maximum dose. The meds are working well. It is such a relief. I didn't realise how much I had struggled mightily to live a functional, successful life. No more inner battles and torment. I see myself as being on meds for life. And I am so glad for this.

The bottom line is this:

Many people are wary about getting an ADHD diagnosis or label. It doesn't matter what label you have. The label doesn't define who you are. It defines your symptoms. If the ADHD meds works, then who cares what label you have. The most important thing is that you can have a better quality of life. You only have one life, why should your life be harder just because you have ADHD?

Parents tell me that they are not giving their child ADHD medication. Please consider the following fact. If your child has type 1 diabetes, this means that the body doesn't produce the hormone insulin. Without that, the body can't properly get the energy and fuel it needs from glucose. Your child needs a daily insulin injection. Preventing this treatment is cruel and life threatening.

If your child has ADHD, they have a deficiency in dopamine and norepinephrine. ADHD is a physical condition, just like type 1 diabetes. Administering the ADHD meds has been found to increase the dopamine levels in the brain and improve the attention in those with ADHD.

ADHD is a physical condition just like type 1 diabetes. The meds work. If your child has it, you owe it to your child to try it out and see the difference. If you have ADHD, you owe it to yourself to try it out and see the difference it can make in your life. If one type of medication doesn't work, don't give up. Just try another one until you experience change. Then you can decide if you will take the meds long-term.

There is so much ignorance surrounding ADHD even among the medical world. Two psychiatrists, one NHS and one private recently told me that the ADHD meds helps for ALL of the ADHD symptoms. The meds do not help for all of ADHD. When working well, it helps for up to 70%. The rest is alternative therapies such as ADHD coaching, which gives you the skills that your brain is lacking.

The ADHD meds is not magic, but it when working properly, and successfully, is as close to magic as you can get. It doesn't help me with my working memory deficit, which is crippling. But it helps with enough of my ADHD symptoms to be worth taking long-term. The ADHD symptoms change with age. They often worsen as women get older. Many undiagnosed ADHD women between the ages of 40 and 55, are suffering so badly, unnecessarily.

I have achieved the impossible with my ADHD, instilling routines and ADHD friendly changes in my life and the life of my family, and helping countless clients to manage their ADHD successfully. Currently, the meds help me to continue along my path with more ease. I no longer feel that I am fighting against myself. Life is hard enough, why should my life be harder than it already is?

Why should the meds only be prescribed for those who are not doing well with their ADHD?

I feel so empowered. So many challenges that I have gone

through in my life now make sense. My dad died when I was a young child. I am an only child, which is very unusual in my circles. I don't have siblings to compare myself to, but I have many cousins to compare to. My mum always said that my dad could never keep down a job. He smoked his whole life. He spread happiness wherever he went. (All point to possible undiagnosed ADHD).

I have been told off for sharing this information, I may damage my family's reputation. There are two types are people in this world, the leaders and the followers. These comments are usually made by those who have not yet accepted their role in life. I am a leader. I lead, not by direction, I lead by personal example. My story has helped countless people find their direction in their lives. In my small way, I have made this world a better place.

MANAGING ANXIETY

My unexplained very high anxiety when I was young, now fits in. Now that the meds are working, I am much calmer. My anxiety was mainly caused/made worse by my unmanaged ADHD. By those chemicals in the brain that were unbalanced. My intense nature, my high and low moods, well this is a common characteristic associated with ADHD. Now my moods are more evenly balanced.

Now that I am on the meds, when problems come up, I handle them CALMLY! And don't turn into a drama queen…

I own my impulsivity, that inner feeling that pushes me to push bravely on and do things that other people just wouldn't do to forward my ADHD career so that I can help more women with ADHD access their potential, my pioneering spirit, my foresight and vision. You see these are the strengths of my ADHD. I own them.

WHAT COMES FIRST, AN ADHD DIAGNOSIS, OR ADHD SKILLS?

There are many paths that lead to the top of the mountain. It doesn't matter which path you choose, as long as you stay on that path. In an ideal world getting your ADHD diagnosis and meds would be ideal. Then you can learn the ADHD tools that you need to live your successful ADHD life. Life doesn't always work out the way you want it to.

Just focus on staying on that mountain. Most of my clients do not have an ADHD diagnosis, and are doing just fine. I wish my clients would ask me before they sign up for a private ADHD assessment. Many private ADHD psychiatrists do not give proper ADHD assessments and even less aftercare, which is what you need. All that money spent…when they could have gotten better service with another private psychiatrist.

If you think that you will wait and first get your ADHD diagnosis before starting ADHD coaching, this may just be magical (perfectionistic) thinking…The only time to start is right now.

If you have been prescribed ADHD meds and they are not working, or you don't have regular contact with your prescriber, you may be experiencing patient neglect. Sadly, this is a very common scenario in the UK, even with private practitioners. You need to make your doctor work harder for you. The meds really can help you manage your ADHD.

FOREWORD - PROFESSOR SUSAN YOUNG

ADHD is a complex condition, not only because it is associated with high rates of comorbidity but because it affects a person in multiple areas of their everyday functioning – in how they interact with family, friends and colleagues; how they perform at school, college or work, and the type of interests they develop and how they spend their time. I first started working with adults with ADHD when I set up the psychology service at the Maudsley Hospital Adult ADHD Service in 1994. In those days, this was a national service and over the years I have seen first-hand the uphill struggle of young people and adults to gain recognition of the condition and receive appropriate treatments. We now have international guidelines about the diagnosis, treatment and management of people with ADHD throughout their life span.

There is increasing evidence for a care approach incorporating both psychopharmacological treatment and psychological treatment as this has been associated with superior outcome than one intervention alone. As such, a multimodal approach should be promoted in the treatment of ADHD but the challenge has been to develop psychotherapeutic treatments that are effective in reducing functional outcomes associated with ADHD. Importantly, these interventions should also aim to foster the hope and belief that the person has the potential to achieve and improve their quality of life.

Unfortunately, many people with ADHD have a sad story to tell and their future seems bleak. The negative outcomes of ADHD are well documented and because of that it comes with a stigma, which is obstructive. We all want to feel pride in what we do, and to feel valued by others, and what I like about this self-help book is that it focuses on the positive – how an individual can identify and build on their strengths in order to create new windows of opportunity and improve quality of life. It is my firm belief that 'pills do not build skills' and this is where coaching techniques are of value because they provide discrete solution-focused methods that support an individual to manage the challenges they face and guide them to achieve successful outcomes in their daily activities. Peppered with interesting vignettes, the book is highly accessible to the reader. In 'user friendly' language, it provides a psychoeducational focus that demystifies 'executive dysfunction' and its relationship with ADHD. The book adopts a pragmatic approach with goal-directed steps that will encourage and motivate the reader to succeed by maximizing their strengths as well as acquiring techniques to overcome their weaknesses. It addresses how to deal with potential obstacles to achievement, such as procrastination, which is the culprit that often interferes with a person's ability to start projects, and/or their motivation to complete them. I congratulate Faigy on this useful book. It is an important addition to the self-help ADHD toolbox.

Susan Young
www.psychology-services.uk.com

ACKNOWLEDGEMENTS

I would like to thank my husband and children for their patience and belief in me. I would like to thank the supportive team who helped this book reach you. I am indebted to the wonderful team of mentors at the Manchester branch of the Digital Google Garage for their invaluable support and advice over the past 3 years. I would like to thank the various professionals who contributed towards this book; Rupinder Howard for her valuable advice; Dr. Art O. Malley for his expert feedback.

MY BOOK JOURNEY

Writing this book has been a life transforming journey. The idea came to me simply because more needs to be done in the UK to address the misconceptions and pervasive ignorance surrounding ADHD. Around two years ago I experienced some frustrating moments regarding educating schools, being informed by a few schools that there was currently no child in their school that had ADHD. I felt like I was up against a brick wall, in my local community and in the wider national community.

I had a thought one morning, about how frustrating my work is on a daily basis. As the lone ambassador for ADHD in my local community, my job of educating the public is not easy. How could I stand by when children and teens suffered simply due to ignorance? There is so much work to be done nationwide to help create the proper awareness around ADHD.

I heard an inner voice, my soul voice that gave me no rest, urgently telling me that I must do more to decrease the stigma here in the UK around ADHD and to increase ADHD awareness and spread appropriate knowledge and ADHD tools. I decided to write a book to demystify ADHD. I jumped in with true ADHD impulsivity and enthusiasm without thinking too much about the challenges that would lie ahead…I opened my laptop and got started.

I see clearly the humbling journey that G-d has led me on, leading me to meet the right people at the right time, and finding out about important information relating to my book. This has given me the strength to move forwards towards completing this book.

I wear two hats, I am an ADHD coach and ADHD coach trainer, and an ADHD parent. When my children were young, and I was going through those terribly dark years of uncertainty, loneliness and worry, I wish that someone would have handed a book to me that explained ADHD in understandable terms, and that had some practical strategies.

This book is my personal gift to my younger self.

I believe that success means action, the results from one's success come from G-d. This book is a success simply because I have had a dream, I have acted on it, and I have *completed* it to the (bittersweet) end. The results are out of my control. This book's project has been my life mission over the past year. Writing this book has been a roller-coaster ride. It has been an exhilarating, and terrifying experience. I have forced myself to move way out my comfort zone in ways that I could never have imagined. It has been so inspiring to meet the many wonderful people who have helped to shape this book.

I believe that the only thing to fear is fear itself. I have pushed through because I know that this book will help you and countless people in turn transform their lives.

The most difficult part of writing a book is knowing when it is finished. The most important part is to finish it in a 'good enough' state, and get it published. So here it is.

PREFACE

Welcome.

Although we have never met, I know you quite well. You see, as you and I are both members of the human race, we have each experienced personal life challenges. Our outer challenges may be unique however we share similar inner struggles. The more I travel through life the more I see that there is more that bonds people than separates them.

Do the following questions reflect some of your inner challenges?

QUESTION	YES	NO
Are you spending too much time covering up your inconsistencies and failings to family and friends?		
Have you been very successful in the past, only to blow it all?		
Do you sense that you possess creative talents but have no clue how to unlock your potential?		
When you are with others do you feel that you are different in some way but can't figure out how?		
Do you feel like you are riding an emotional roller coaster?		
Are you ashamed of the lies (read excuses) that you have created to cover up your incompetencies?		
Do you shift from being super motivated to totally unmotivated?		
Have you failed so many times that you don't trust yourself anymore?		
Is your mind racing with multiple		

thoughts competing for your attention?		
Can you sometimes focus intently for long periods of time but other times you have great difficulty focusing?		
Would you love to find out how you can create your true calm and inner peace?		
Do you feel that you are always running after time?		
Do you crave organisation but don't know how to get there?		
Do you feel an internal block is preventing you from reaching your potential no matter how hard you try?		
Do you sense that you have been putting in far more effort than your peers to reach your goals with less than remarkable results?		
Have you no idea what your life goals should be?		
Would you love to know how to overcome your challenges and reach your success?		

If you have answered, 'yes' to most of these questions then read on. This book is for creative, talented people just like yourself. It addresses your problems head-on and offers simple practical solutions that will lead you swiftly towards your success.

You *can* stop the negative cycle of despair and hopelessness. You *can* achieve long lasting positivity and permanent inner change.

You possess enormous talent. How do I know this? This world was created perfectly balanced. If you are experiencing major inner challenges, you must also possess great inner strengths. You possess unique qualities in a combination and strength that no one from the beginning of time until the very end of time will ever possess. Your deficits are simply a smoke screen obscuring a wonderfully gifted you. Through reading this book I hope that you will start to pay more attention to those strengths. The more you start to focus on them, the more they will develop.

Please stop being ashamed of your ADHD. Your ADHD is a powerful gift that has been given to you by G-d. ADHD stands for Attention Deficit Hyperactivity Disorder.

In my work as an ADHD coach, I see the shame, confusion, and humiliation that my clients have faced their entire lives. I see the loss of self-esteem and self-confidence that once lost, is so hard to build up. I see the untold damage that this has done to them. Your ADHD is not a disease, and is not caused by bad parenting or laziness.

I love my work because I help my clients focus on and develop their strengths.

The way forward is to understand that your ADHD is not your fault, you were born like this. Your ADHD is a gift. The way forward is to start to focus on your strengths, and use them to serve you in your life mission.

It is time to understand your ADHD, take ownership of it, and unlock your strengths. Time to climb out of your head and live and succeed inside your body.

This book first delves into the brain's executive functions and how they have an impact in your life. Then you will understand about your ADHD and the different types of treatment. There is a strengths and challenges chart at the back of the book. Use it to gain greater self-awareness, and thereby greater potential for change.

It is well known that the world's best coaches are those who have been through their personal dark times and then found their personal light. I have lived with the challenges of time management, internal disorganisation, and ADHD dysfunction in various forms for most of my life. I have had my dark times. Times that have forced me to search for the light.

It has been one of the hardest tasks I have ever done. I I

have created myself anew in the process and learnt some great coping strategies. My internal challenges are all still present, but I have the necessary skills to compensate for, and overcome them. I can honesty testify that due to my internal work over the last 20 years, I now live the dream ADHD life. I know that you can do this for your life.

My personal vision is to make a significant contribution to the world based on my own experiences and training. I bring to you my belief in your ability to change and to move forward to reach your goals.

This book is an overview about ADHD. It addresses readers who already have an ADHD diagnosis, or those who strongly suspect they may have ADHD.

The insights, tips and anecdotes included within this book are my gift to you, to empower you. Understanding the root of your struggles leads to ownership and self-acceptance, which brings motivation and action in turn.

In the UK, very few people with ADHD manage to access the available help, (more about that later in the book). ADHD is still very much seen as something to hide. This problematic attitude is a huge barrier for accessing the vital tools that you require to get your life back on track.

It is my dream that soon, ADHD will become widely understood for what it is and the shame and stigma surrounding it will disappear. The purpose of this book is to guide and support you along your journey of inner discovery. It is designed to expand your awareness and make you think.

Your ADHD is a massive strength, when harnessed correctly can bring you more success than you ever dreamed of. Most of my clients start coaching, focusing on their weaknesses. They don't even believe that they have strengths. Their deficits act as a smoke screen covering up their strengths. It is my fervent wish that you will start to uncover your strengths and start to focus more on them.

Your ADHD challenges are not your fault, and you need not suffer alone. It is your responsibility to go and take advantage of the available guidance. Your strengths are uniquely yours. Use them to help you overcome your ADHD challenges and in doing so you will unlock the door to your life success.

The ideas in this book are all based on hard facts and clear evidence. Please note, you will not find all the answers that you are looking for in this book. It is intended to jump start you along your journey of self-understanding. When you have finished reading this book if you have more questions than before you started, then this book will have served its purpose.

If you have more questions, I would love to hear from you. Contact me at: faigy@focuswithfaigy.com

ACHIEVE SUCCESS AND STOP WASTING YOUR TIME

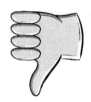

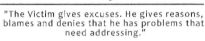

"The Victor gets results. He takes ownership, accountability and responsibility for his challenges."

"The Victim gives excuses. He gives reasons, blames and denies that he has problems that need addressing."

Think of an imaginary line stretching horizontally across this page.

There are two groups of people – those that live above the line and those below it. Those above the line take 'ownership' for their problems, take on the 'responsibility' to reach their actions, and are 'accountable' for their solutions. They are the ones who reach their goals, having faced their failures and pain head on. They succeed because in this world, hard work (and prayer) usually pays off.

The second group lives below the line. They 'blame' themselves and others for their problems. They give 'excuse's why they haven't reached their goals, or why they can't meet their deadlines. They 'deny' having a problem in the first place. They are the victims of the world, often miserable and bitter. They get nowhere in life.

It is part of the human condition to shift above and below the line. As you read this book, you will encounter new ideas. You may witness an internal resistance. Simply observe yourself, and gently bring yourself back above the line.

Some ideas in this book may be easy to implement, others may seem difficult at first. If you find yourself resisting a new idea, simply observe yourself. Where is this coming from? If you approach the ideas with a curious, open mind, and a willingness to try them out, you will succeed. If you come across an idea and it doesn't appeal to you, simply put it in your back pocket for later use. You never know when you might want to retrieve it.

You may already be familiar with many of the ideas presented in this book. To get the most out of it, keep an open and curious 'above-the-line' mindset. Replace, "I know this idea already," with, "How can I take this familiar idea and deepen my understanding?"

When you make a conscious choice to address your challenges, the universe reacts according to your choice and actions.

It may not be easy to carry out some of the exercises. You may encounter fear or pain. Be kind and understanding to yourself. Push through little by little until you will find yourself in a better place.

Long-term habit change takes time. If you want to improve your executive functions, you need to choose a very small goal. You need to be committed 200% and willing to stick to your goal without distractions for a while.

So many of my clients want to see major life altering results, yesterday. When this doesn't happen, they get frustrated, demotivated, and quit. When this occurs, they are worse off than before they started!

Choose a really small goal, stick to it no matter what. Each small step will take you slowly but surely towards your goal.

PART 2
YOUR POWER TOOL KIT

YOUR EXECUTIVE FUNCTIONS

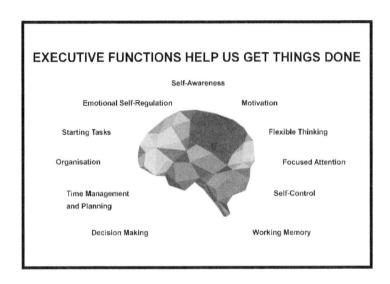

EXECUTIVE FUNCTIONS HELP US GET THINGS DONE

Self-Awareness

Emotional Self-Regulation · Motivation

Starting Tasks · Flexible Thinking

Organisation · Focused Attention

Time Management and Planning · Self-Control

Decision Making · Working Memory

Consider the following questions:

- Have you noticed that some people possess great talents yet surprisingly do not reach their potential?
- Do you know people of average or below average intelligence who have gone far in life?
- Can you honestly say that you have tried harder than your peers at school/college and beyond, and you have still had disappointing results in relation to your efforts?

You were born with all the skills necessary to reach your own version of success. These skills are located in the front of your brain, in the pre-frontal cortex, directly behind your forehead. They are called your executive functions. You will learn more about your executive functions and how they play a vital role in your life success, in the next few parts of this book.

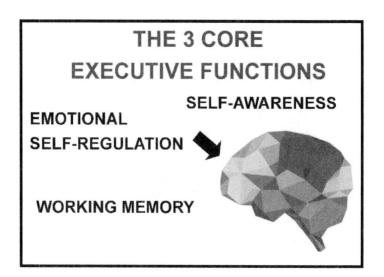

THE 3 CORE
EXECUTIVE FUNCTIONS

SELF-AWARENESS

EMOTIONAL
SELF-REGULATION

WORKING MEMORY

The three core executive functions are:

1. Your self-awareness
2. Your level of emotional self-regulation
3. Your working memory

These three executive function skills are the driving force behind your actions. They are interconnected like junctions in a complex road system. The other executive function skills (roads) have to pass through these three junctions to work at their optimum level. When you work on these three executive functions, you should see noticeable change in the other executive functions.

The next executive function skills are:

1. Your focus powers
2. Your organisation skills
3. Your procrastination and motivation level
4. Your life adaptability
5. Your decision and prioritising skills
6. Your time management and planning skills

7.   Your level of self-control

More about the above executive functions later in the book. Before you get overwhelmed that there is simply far too much to work on, please understand that when you work on one area consistently, you will see change in other areas. I see this daily with my clients. This is because all the executive functions are interconnected. When one improves, the other functions improve as well.

No one in this world has the perfect brain. There will be some skills that you naturally possess in abundance, and some you need to work on. You will possess some of every trait.

When you see a beautiful, strong tree you know that the roots are healthy. Your executive functions are the roots of your tree, the roots of your life. Those who seem to be high achievers, who get so much done in their day, and handle challenges with focused calm, simply have sturdier roots and better executive function skills than you.

The good news is that if your executive function tools are not internally developed, you can strengthen them with external tools.

There is a lot of overlap between the different executive functions. As you progress through this book you will understand how each executive function work together and are linked and work together.

According to leading ADHD researcher Dr. Russell Barkley, the average person's executive functions are only fully developed at around the age of thirty. If you have ADHD your executive functions may never fully develop, hence your challenges. You may need tools to support your executive functions for life. *Since the executive functions are all linked, when you work on one executive function trait you should see an improvement in other executive functions.*

You can be as intelligent as Einstein, but if your talents are not contained within the vessel of healthy executive functions, they will be irrelevant and useless. It is vital for your life success that you build a strong vessel to contain your wonderful creative talents and strengths. The more you work on developing your executive functions, the more you will achieve.

Your executive functions are your 'power-tool-kit' and when you understand how to channel your executive functions, they will hold hands and form a circle of power and energy surrounding and supporting you.

There is no single consensus regarding the definition of executive functions. I have based my interpretation on the model by psychologists Peg Dawson, Ed.D., and Richard Guare, Ph.D.

WHO DISCOVERED THE EXECUTIVE FUNCTION CONCEPT?

Executive functions became more widely recognised in the 1970s. Professionals treating ADHD patients realised that people with head injuries to the pre-frontal lobes showed similar symptoms to those with ADHD, (Lezak 1979). It was discovered that ADHD is a brain-based developmental condition. Many studies have been conducted over the years that verify this. (Singh, et al. 2015). ADHD is a medical condition, just like any other medical condition. In brain scans parts of the ADHD brain are different.

The medical world is constantly making advances in understanding executive functions. There is now consensus among mental health practitioners that ADHD is itself an executive function developmental deficit (Barkley, 2010). This means that if you have ADHD you will have executive function deficit. *You can have executive function deficit without having ADHD.* This book addresses those who have ADHD and also those who just have some executive function deficit.

If your executive function deficits are consistently holding you back, so that you feel that there is a hidden block that is stopping you from succeeding in life, then it is time to learn some tools to support your executive function deficit.

SELF-AWARENESS

Your height, which is biological, will develop on its own. Self-awareness, and the other executive function skills mentioned in this book will also develop on their own, but only up to a certain point. After this point of development, you will need to learn tools to improve your self-awareness, and implement strategies to help you manage successfully in your life.

The level of your self-awareness will determine the level of your executive functions. Your self-awareness is the key to your success and happiness. It is about paying attention to your own thinking.

Self-awareness is like having two people perched on your shoulder, the angel and the devil. They are constantly talking to you, guiding you how to act and solve problems. Self-awareness is the voice inside your head that is constantly talking to you about the choices you make.

Pay attention to that internal dialogue. What volume is it set to? If you are struggling in certain areas, one voice may be set too low. In many cases it may be on mute. This is one cause why you feel stuck in some areas in your life. Many of my clients relate how their 'devil' voice, or inner critic is set way to high.

Self-awareness is about thinking about your thinking. Just like the stick figure in the drawing who is thinking about his thinking. When you are in a difficult situation, how easily can you at that moment mentally come out of yourself, 'perch yourself on your shoulder' look down at the situation and guide yourself.

If you can do this, then you have excellent self-awareness skills. You are most likely successful in many areas of your life. If you find this difficult, then learning tools to help you increase your self-awareness is vital to your life success.

When I start to work with a new client, they often have lots of big lofty goals. I show them how to break down those goals into one goal, self-awareness. If they can improve their level of self-awareness in relation to that goal, they will be well on the way to their success. Self-awareness is like the engine in your car. The size and make of your car are irrelevant. The more powerful your engine, the faster your car will go.

> Eric was 19 and still living at home. He started coaching to learn coping strategies. As his first commitment to change, he renewed his gym membership to help manage his ADHD. His mum wanted him to fund his gym membership. He called me in a panic. He couldn't afford to pay for gym membership. He was really upset and believed there was no solution. I simply asked him to think about alternative, free exercise options. He couldn't come up with any ideas. I suggested jogging as an alternative exercise. He committed to two sessions of 15 minutes each week. I asked him to start on that very day and let me know how he got on. At the next session, he related that he had jogged four times for over an hour each time.

As soon as Eric felt stuck his internal dialogue disappeared. I stepped in to act as his inner voice, guiding him towards a solution. If you have developed good self-awareness skills you will be able to come up with the solution to your problems *by yourself.*

The 'silenced mind' is the source of many impulsive actions. Think back to a time when you got angry or lost control in some way. At that time, your mind's voice disappeared just when you needed it most to guide you through the situation.

Current research shows, that if you have ADHD it will

take you a long time to learn from previous mistakes (Barkley, 2010). I have personally seen this pattern with many of my clients. You may be making the same mistakes repeatedly until you finally see a pattern, and hopefully change your course of action. This is due in large part to your malfunctioning mind-voice.

Sarah was asked to make some of her famous chocolate mousse cups for the village fair. She related how frustrated she was with herself that it took her until cup number eight to realise that she should adjust the pouring angle so the mousse wouldn't spill over onto the counter. She observed her silenced mind's voice in action. A loud mind's voice would have guided her towards success far earlier than the eighth cup.

How can you raise the volume? Simply bring in that voice from an external source. Talk to yourself out loud! This may not sound very conventional, but it works! Countless clients have reported amazing success through using this simple tool.

The next time you are faced with a dilemma; pause and imagine yourself looking down onto yourself from a bird's eye view. Guide yourself by verbalising the different options available *out loud.*

Have you ever told someone that you just need them to listen as you process your thoughts? You may be doing this already without even realising it.

Greta didn't understand why she couldn't stay focused on her studies. Her mum was at her wits end. They both knew that if she failed her exams she would not get into the university of her choice. Greta learned to use her inner mind's voice as a tool to help her get started, stay focused and most importantly, finish off her work. She started to talk out loud to herself to motivate herself to start tasks, and stay on task. She was hesitant at first, but after seeing significant results she was delighted. She adapted this method to other areas of her life. She found that she was finally able to get up on time in the mornings, something she hadn't managed in years.

When Claire had a chocolate craving, she would catch herself, and loudly say, "You don't need that chocolate bar. It's bad for you." She was astounded to see that she was able to control herself. She increased her self-awareness by identifying certain times of the day when she was prone to daydreaming and wasting time. She started talking out loud to herself to hurry up and move on. It really worked!

Angela understood the dangers of poor self-awareness very well. Her Mum, an otherwise kind, upstanding woman suffered from poor self-awareness in certain areas. Her mum was unaware how her anxiety and lack of patience were eating away at her personal and family life. These behaviours had gone on for over forty years. Angela had grown up with them. She was terrified of subconsciously perpetuating similar behaviours with her own family. She went for therapy to help her work through her fears and trauma.

YOUR WORKING MEMORY

Working memory is the second of the three core executive function skills that directly impact the efficiency of all the other skills.

Here are just some of the different types of memory.

1. Working memory
2. Auditory processing
3. Short-term memory
4. Long-term memory
5. Spatial memory
6. Prospective memory

WORKING MEMORY

Working memory is the part of your thinking process where you keep track of the information you need right now. It is like your mental notepad. It is the ability to hold information in your mind, and manipulate it in order to complete complex tasks such as reasoning, learning and comprehension, even amidst distractions. It is the ability to carry out a conversation even when there is lots of noise and distractions going on. If you can remember multi-step directions without having to write them down, then you have excellent working memory skills.

If you forget mid-conversation what you were going to say, or often forget what you were going to do next, rest assured that you are not losing your mind. You simply have a poor working memory, and you are observing it in action.

Since your working memory is one of the three core executive functions if you have a poor working memory, you will naturally have many more challenges with the other executive functions such as organisation, time management and planning.

AUDITORY PROCESSING

This function is directly connected with your working memory. If you have a malfunctioning working memory you may find yourself misunderstanding information that has been given to you more often than you care to admit. Do find it difficult to focus and process what is being said to you? This may be a sign that you have poor auditory processing skills.

Emily went on holiday with her three children. Her husband had booked the homebound train tickets for her. He was travelling by car, taking the suitcases with him. Emily was standing at the station with her children, and was surprised that the train she was supposed to catch just sailed by without stopping. She looked at her ticket again and realised in horror that she was at the wrong station. For the last two weeks her husband had mentioned a different station and she had misheard him, misreading the information on the ticket, and booking the taxi to take her and her children to the wrong station...

Imagine her feelings of incompetence and shame, her emotional turmoil, and the stress and humiliation of having to purchase new train tickets. What impact did this have on her marriage and her self-trust?

SHORT-TERM MEMORY

When you learn something new, your brain first stores it in your short-term memory bank, and then transfers it to your long-term memory for easy retrieval. You might be learning a new topic, or taking instructions from your boss, and it all makes sense at the time. Then later in the day, you can't remember any of it. Do you suffer from that dizzy, floating feeling? These challenges are simply your impaired working memory in action. This can really hold you back in life.

LONG-TERM MEMORY

This is the ability to store information into your long-term memory bank so that when you need the information you can access it easily. Some people have excellent long-term memory, and poor short-term memory, and vice versa. How easily can you recall information that has been stored from the past like people's names and birthdays? When you need to recall a memory, do you sense that your brain takes longer to bring up the information that is stored in your long-term memory bank?

SPATIAL MEMORY

Spatial memory is the ability to record information about your environment. If you have a good spatial memory you can easily remember where you left your phone or where you have placed those important documents, even when there are a lot of other distractions going on in your environment.

Amanda wasted a lot of money with her clothing purchases. She really wanted to be more careful. However, she felt that there was an inner enemy sabotaging her efforts, no matter how hard she tried. Why was she constantly losing those purchase receipts? Was there something wrong with her vision? Was she losing her mind? She would pay for an item and watch with her own eyes how the cashier placed the receipt into the bag. Yet when she wanted to return the item, the receipt had either vanished into thin air or she had placed the wrong receipt together with the item.

Elaine was a mother of two primary school aged children. The end of the academic school year was approaching. She had always thought it would be a nice gesture to write thank you cards to her children's teachers, but had not yet managed to do so. This year, she wanted to make a real effort to give a thoughtful present and card. She had bought everything she needed. The night before, the last day of school, Elaine couldn't find the lovely cards she had bought. Pre-coaching she would have eaten herself up over this, berating herself for her stupidity. Post-coaching, Elaine understood that she was only human. She understood that her working memory was at fault. She actually saw the humour in the moment. She briefly searched for the cards. When she couldn't find them, she simply wrote the cards on simple white paper without any self-recrimination. She spent an extra minute writing thoughtfully and presented the notes to the teachers with her head held high.

PROSPECTIVE MEMORY

You may also have a poor 'prospective memory'. This is the ability to plan for the future, and remember details or events that will happen in the future. It is the ability to independently break down the tasks so you can easily plan to reach your goals. (Fuermaier, et al. 2013). You may be living in the 'now and the not now' in life, and you may find it very difficult to plan ahead for events that haven't yet occurred.

Experts have found a great way to support your prospective memory is to act out your future goals. Acting out information or future actions makes it easier to recall them and implement plans of action when needed. (Jaroslawska, et al. 2016).

THE WORKING MEMORY TABLE

There is another way to explain working memory. Imagine it as a small table that can only hold four items or ideas at once. Have you ever had that maddening experience of entering a room and promptly forgetting what you came in for? As you entered the room new sensory data entered your brain, pushing off an old piece of information that was on your working memory table, in order to accommodate the new one. If you are not actively engaged in a thought it will fall off your table and get replaced by another thought. If this happens on a daily basis it can be very frustrating. It can really hold you back.

Working memory usually improves with age. On average, children under five years of age can hold one or two items in their working memory. Over age five they can hold three or four pieces of information. Your working memory becomes fully functional at around age 25. (Executive Function Success). At this age if you have a good working memory you can hold up to seven items at a time in your consciousness. However, if you have a working memory deficit, there will be a limit to its development. The level of your working memory

OWN YOUR ADHD

may permanently be lagging behind your peers.

Peter's 11-year-old daughter, Tabitha was training to become a professional dancer. The course was divided into two parts. The first part was creative dancing, which she excelled in. The second part followed a complicated routine of steps. Tabitha's teacher couldn't understand why she became so agitated and upset. She had daily meltdowns. She just couldn't follow the routine. Tabitha was assessed and diagnosed with ADD. Subsequently, when her teacher broke the steps down into small bite size chunks she managed them beautifully. Her working memory was supported, and she went on to win many awards.

Test the level of your working memory. Repeat a list of words in alphabetical order and say them *in reverse.* How many did you remember, in order? This exercise is designed to help you witness your own working memory in action. It is very difficult to improve your working memory. You can use external supports to guide you. You will need to repeat things to yourself out loud, and carry a notepad and pen around with you *everywhere.* As you go about your day and meet new people, jot down important information. Designate a home for your notebook when you're not using it. Doing this will help combat that horrible floating feeling and keep you grounded.

A great way to support your working memory is to set up routines as much as possible. With my clients I have seen how much they have benefitted from this. When you need to remember what to do next, this taxes your thinking (working memory) space, and causes unnecessary stress. By automating your actions, you free up precious head space for other more important activities, (Child Mind Institute 2018).

Too many of my clients tell me that they have emotional problems and mistakenly think that they need therapy. This may be true but if they have a smaller working memory table, in some cases only being able to hold 2 or less pieces of information at a time, then this will have a massive impact on their wellbeing, focus and inner peace and of course their life productivity.

Therapy won't fix your working memory deficit. Therapy will be necessary to repair the emotional damage that has happened as a result of your unsupported working memory deficit tripping you up in your life. Clients have found that simply by supporting their working memory deficit they feel calmer and more focused, and they don't even need therapy after all.

Many clients tell me that they work slowly. They find it difficult to multi-task. One source for this is the working memory deficit. They can only hold one piece of information in the forefront of their mind. Your working memory level will stay for life. There is not much you can do to improve it. You can simply need to learn tools to support your working memory deficit. When you do so successfully then your efficiency will improve.

EMOTIONAL SELF-REGULATION

Your emotional barometer is the third executive function that you need for your focus and success.
Consider the following questions:

- When you get depressed, angry or anxious does it take a long time (hours or even days) to get back to your normal state?
- In that time frame does your productivity level dip dramatically?
- When you get back to yourself, do you have to pick up the pieces?
- Do you tend towards bursts of flash anger?
- Do you have trouble remembering the lead up to your outburst?
- Do you get anxious or depressed, and can't seem to shake off your negative feelings?
-

These tendencies may be signs of emotional dysregulation. This means that your feelings may easily swing between positive and negative, and that comes in the way of your life success. When 'life happens' when you encounter a problem, or you have a 'win' in your life, how far do your emotions swing? How easily do you get thrown off balance by your emotions, and what effect does this have on your life? When that happens, become notice (become more self-aware) what happens to the levels of your focus and productivity.

The executive function trait of emotional self-regulation is like a bully. It takes over your brain when you least expect it. Your day can be running so well, your executive functions may be working efficiently, then something happens that throws you off balance. You get upset, and all your executive functions shut down. You become stuck, overwhelmed, and can't move on even if you desperately want to (Matthies, et al.

2016). This is the heart of your ADHD challenge.

> Alan was in coaching for six months. I sensed that his intense emotional volatility was an area he would specifically benefit from working on. I waited until he was ready to address it. One day, during a session he had a verbal meltdown, an extreme reaction to an innocent comment that I had made. I simply listened until he had finished.
>
> It wasn't easy to listen to him. He ranted for a full twenty minutes without stopping, venting his frustrations out on me. When he was spent, he became really upset that he had wasted the session, and most importantly gotten upset. When he calmed down, he simply couldn't recall what had triggered his reaction.
>
> I calmly informed him that this session had been the most productive one to date. He finally saw how much his emotional impulsivity was getting in the way, and he was now ready to address it.

Let's explore why this happens. Your brain was designed to protect you, but sometimes the protection mechanism malfunctions. Your limbic system located in your brain, acts as your security guard, protecting you from danger. If you see a dangerous animal walking towards you, or realise that you are overdue with a project for your boss, your limbic system rapidly moves into high alert.

It cannot differentiate between these two rather different scenarios. It just senses the negative feelings of fear, anxiety or worry, and jumps in to protect you. Where you allow your feelings to lead you from here is a good indicator of how successful you will be in all areas of your life.

You will either become super angry (fight), run away from your situation by distracting yourself (flight), or become overwhelmed and paralysed, (freeze).

Your brain gravitates towards one or two types of protective behaviour. Recognising your coping mechanism is the first step towards change. (This is self-awareness). When you feel stuck understand that your mind voice has packed its bags and out for lunch. With a few tricks you can coax it back.

Ellen was a new organising client. 20 minutes before our second session her husband texted that she was feeling unwell and had to cancel. At our next session I asked her how she was feeling. "I had so much to do, and I just couldn't handle it. I went to bed and stayed there for two days until I felt better." A typical flight and freeze reaction to stress.

If you have ADHD or challenges with your executive functions, you must understand that you may experience *both positive and negative* emotions more intensely. You may sense that you get very excitable and enthusiastic, perhaps more than your peers. Please understand that you have a powerful gift. You have the potential to experience the richness of life on a far deeper level than other people. Your negative feelings may be stopping you from accessing your wonderful emotional gifts.

Let's focus on some common emotional challenges that are common, especially if you have ADHD.

RUMINATION

Do you have a loud internal critic that accompanies you wherever you go? This is your internal enemy! When you get upset do you focus on your thoughts so intently that your thoughts paralyse your functioning? When you are bored does this intensify? Research has proven what we have known for a long time. Many people are born with a genetic pre-disposition towards negative thinking. Your mind processes over 70,000 thoughts every day. If you are predisposed towards negative thinking patterns then that is a huge dose of daily negativity that you are facing.

Your ADHD brain craves entertainment and stimulation. It can't cope with boredom, and will zone in on any available distraction in an attempt to entertain itself. Where there is a vacuum, negativity quickly fills the space. *Your brain might even lure you into a negative thought cycle just to keep itself occupied and entertained.* This is a major contributing factor why you find it difficult to get boring tasks done.

The only way out is to increase your self-awareness. Become aware of your thoughts and stop them in their tracks as soon as you can, before they take root. Replace them with positive ones as soon as possible.

Changing your environment is a great way to stop or lessen the negative pull. Go for a walk or meet up with a friend. These strategies are most effective when the negative thought process is caught at an early stage.

Angela's inner critic constantly pulverised her for her incompetency. Today it was, "Why did you leave food out on the counter the entire night? Lazy slob, now the food's spoiled." Angela understood that her brain gravitated away from boring tasks and, well, packing away the food was boring and even painful. There were too many details to think about, the fridge needed organising before she could fit in any more food. There were too many steps to focus on. It took time, but she learned to recognise her internal critic and to respond appropriately to maintain her emotional balance.

Talk back to your inner critic. Talk out loud! It may sound daft, but who cares? It works! When you start to talk back to your inner critic you weaken your inner negative voice, and strengthen your inner positive voice. This is the first step to long- term change. A large part of my work with clients is identifying the inner critic, and the accompanying accusations. We work on creating counter messages to empower and strengthen my clients. They learn to focus on what they are doing right.

Here are a few examples of typical negative thoughts and positive counter thoughts:

"There is only one solution." This type of thinking stems from the 'all or nothing' black and white thought pattern. There are many paths that lead to the top of the mountain.

"No one ever calls me." This is the 'always and never' trap. At this moment in time or on this day no one has called you. It does not mean that no one *ever* calls you.

"My spouse doesn't like me." This is the 'mindreading' trap. It is particularly dangerous in relationships. How do you know your spouse doesn't like you? Just because he/she neglected to do a task does not prove anything.

"It is all someone else's fault." This is your 'blame game' thinking mode. When you blame others, you stay stuck in that mode of thinking and this shuts down avenues of problem solving. You need to accept that you may have contributed to the problem, and look for ways to improve the situation.

"I am a failure." When you blame yourself, you stay firmly stuck in your present situation. Sometimes you may make really stupid mistakes but that is an inevitable part of being human. You are imperfect. Remember that. Find space within yourself to laugh at your mistakes.

"People will laugh at me when I do this." This is your brain lying to you. How do you know the outcome of your actions and other people's reactions? It is likely you will do really well and that people will like what you will do.

"I feel so overwhelmed, I'm going to cancel the commitment." Avoid making a decision based on your feelings. Your feelings are real, but they are not reality! They are a distortion of reality. It is vital to challenge those feelings and acknowledge that they are often a distortion of the truth.

"I forgot my appointment. I *should have* cancelled it in good time." Ban thoughts starting with should/could/must/ought. You are human and you are allowed to make mistakes. This is the best way to learn. Just learn from the incident and move on.

Dwelling on these types of thoughts only pulls you further into the pit of negativity. When you become adept at recognising

OWN YOUR ADHD

negative thoughts, and changing them to positive ones, you will be on your way to overcoming your emotional problems. It can be so difficult to change your thinking patterns. If you persevere, then little by little, day by day, the seemingly small changes will add up.

ARE YOU ASHAMED OF YOUR MISTAKES?

Do you suffer paralysing shame due to your mistakes? Mistakes do not indicate that you are flawed. They are just mistakes, often caused by your executive function challenges. If shame relating to a mistake is a frequent visitor, you will start to validate and internalise your shame (also called 'self-hate'). Over time this will become an entrenched habit.

The first step to overcoming guilt, shame and worry is to acknowledge that your shame is brought about by that loud internal voice that is berating you incessantly. The second step is to understand that no one is perfect, and your mistakes indicate that you are simply a member of the human race.

Below are some positive affirmations that will help you on your journey to overcoming your shameful feelings:

- "I acknowledge my ADHD symptoms."
- "I create my own crises and challenges due to my poor memory recall. I will find solutions to help myself."
- "I process information in a unique way, so I often mishear information. That is OK."
- "My poor time management gets in the way."
- "My disorganisation leads to my own self-made crises. I can create myself anew."

Guilt, shame and worry can become an excuse to continue with your old (familiar and comfortable) behaviour patterns.

To succeed in life, you will need to find a way to forgive yourself and your ADHD deficits.

Julie had difficulties with parking. She related that she had once parked in a multi- storey car park that had very narrow spaces. She had to be guided out of her space by two people. Describing her feelings at the time, she said that she felt split into two separate people observing the scene. One watched the scene unfold in shock and embarrassment. The other was observing in humorous fascination. Julie had a healthy mind-voice, giving balance to both the positive and the negative. She was able to balance the negative feelings of shame with a healthy dose of humour. She made sure to relate this amusing incident to her family in a positive manner, thereby teaching by example that it is perfectly fine to make mistakes, and her mistakes are not a sign of her flawed' personality.

These mistakes will likely repeat themselves will help you plan better for the future. See the humour in your situation. Learn to laugh at your self-made crises. These are often the best teaching moments.

ANXIETY

If you have ADHD, you may be suffering from external and internal stress due to your deficits. To compound the problem, you may well have a secondary anxiety condition, which can worsen if the ADHD symptoms are not addressed. All is not lost. When you get a grip on your executive functions, your anxiety will likely abate.

Fear and anxiety are often intertwined and it may be very difficult to separate the two. Fear is an unpleasant emotion caused by the threat of danger, pain, or harm. Its role is to protect you. Anxiety is excessive worry that can be crippling, often interfering with daily functioning.

Anxiety can be broken down into specific sub-groups:

1. *Phobias* are extreme or irrational fears.
2. *Social phobia* is the fear of situations that involve interaction with other people. You could say social anxiety is the fear and anxiety of being negatively judged and evaluated by other people. The manifestations can be experienced in many areas of a person's life.
3. *Panic disorder* is characterized by sudden episodes of intense fear that trigger severe physical reactions when there is no real danger present. Panic attacks can be very frightening. You might think you're losing control, having a heart attack or even dying.
4. *OCD* is the presence of obsessions, compulsions, or both. Obsessions are defined by recurrent and persistent thoughts, urges or impulses. Compulsions are acts of behaviour that the person feels compelled to do.
5. *GAD* or General Anxiety Disorder is a condition characterised by six months or more of chronic, exaggerated anxiety. People with GAD often expect the worst; they might experience episodes of feeling

lightheaded or out of breath.

If you are suffering from anxiety, it is important to get the help you need as your anxiety will have an impact on your life. Diet, and exercise play a vital role in managing your anxiety, as well as spending time with friends.

ANGER

I believe that ADHD has been misnamed. The term ADHD, meaning, Attention Deficit Hyperactivity Disorder, makes one think that ADHD is a focusing disorder. The fact is that emotional self-disregulation forms the heart of the ADHD challenge. It's the inability to control your emotions, whatever they may be, especially your intense feelings of anger that cause the most trouble for those with ADHD. Anger management issues go hand in hand with ADHD. On one side of the scale you may possess intense energy and enthusiasm. On the other side, you may experience intense feelings of frustration and anger. Flash anger is a particularly debilitating challenge that is associated with your ADHD.

Please understand that if you have ADHD, conventional anger management tools may not work for you. You will need to learn specific strategies to help yourself. The sooner you improve your self-awareness and regain your self-control, the sooner you will see success in your life.

As a general rule, although there are many exceptions. In my clinic I have seen that clients who have ADD (more about that later in the book) tend to suffer more from anxiety and depressive thoughts, while those with ADHD suffer more from anger and anxiety challenges.

Your potential for intense anger is actually a strength. Your anger can be channelled into intense enthusiasm, excitement, motivation and persistence to achieve your goals no matter what. You have a valuable tool that can help you get far in life. Use it to build you, not destroy you.

By increasing your level of self-awareness, you will improve your anger management and your emotional self-regulation.

REJECTION SENSITIVITY DYSPHORIA

If you have ADHD, you may also suffer from RSD or Rejection Sensitivity Dysphoria. This is an intense feeling of being vulnerable when rejected, teased or criticised by the important people in your life. In Greek it means "difficult to bear." If you experience rejection sensitivity, you will feel intense emotional pain to such a degree that it is difficult for you to bear the emotional pain. The emotional pain is experienced as a physical pain. This pain will also be triggered if you sense that you have fallen short of your own expectations. If you experience this intense feeling, you may often feel shame due to your intense emotions. RSD is especially common in women and is a major source of relationship breakdown and divorce among women who have ADHD.

Early childhood trauma can make symptoms worsen over time.

When a person is going through the throes of rejection sensitivity it can look like they have a mood disorder. The sudden change from being perfectly fine to being intensely sad often results in the person being misdiagnosed as having Borderline Personality Disorder, or Bipolar Disorder.

Far too many of my clients, especially women have related how they have been misdiagnosed with Borderline Personality Disorder or Bipolar Disorder, and have been on mood stabilising medications or antidepressants for years, without any follow up. They have reported telling their doctors that the meds doesn't make them feel better yet they are continually prescribed the same medication, often for years on end. Tragically their words are often not taken seriously or even listened to by their practitioners.

ADHD medication usually helps since RSD is often caused by an imbalance of chemicals in the brain. Psychotherapy or CBT usually doesn't help that much, because the emotional reaction overtakes and overwhelms your body and mind very suddenly. Mindfulness is a great tool to manage the non-stop bombarding thoughts that can overtake your mind.

RECOGNITION RESPONSIVE EUPHORIA

If you have ADHD, you may likely have RRE, Recognition Responsive Euphoria. It is even more common than RSD.

If you have ADHD, most likely it went untreated for many years. As a result, you may have made many mistakes, and received more than your fair share of criticism. This has resulted in becoming more excited by the positive recognition when you are praised. If you have ADHD, praise is one of the best ways to motivate you. You must distance yourself from negative people, and surround yourself with genuinely positive people, who recognise your strengths. Use your sensitivity to praise to motivate you to move towards your goals. You have a tremendous power, use it well.

STRESS AND EXECUTIVE FUNCTION DEFICIT

When your executive functions are not working correctly you will experience stress. This will often be in the form of anger, anxiety, overwhelm and fear. While stress is a part of daily life you may be worsening your stressful feelings because of your own self-made crises that arise due to your executive function deficit.

Cortisol, the stress hormone, has been shown to damage and kill cells in the hippocampus, an organ in the brain. There is evidence that chronic stress causes premature brain aging (McEwen, 2007). Recent research has found that it can shorten your life span. It compromises your immune system. Stress is a deadly, silent killer. You owe it to yourself and your family to actively fight it.

When you become stressed, high levels of cortisol flood your brain. To balance this, your brain rapidly releases high levels of norepinephrine and dopamine. This increase in hormones temporarily gives you more strength and keeps you on high alert for danger, when quick reactions are vital. If you are under constant stress however, this defence mechanism can work against you. Those high levels of hormones that are released into your brain start to damage your body.

Do you suffer from the following symptoms? They may be stress related.

Emotional symptoms of stress

- Becoming easily agitated, frustrated or moody
- Feeling overwhelmed; you are losing control or must take control
- Having difficulty relaxing
- Feeling bad about yourself (low self-esteem), feeling lonely, worthless, depressed
- Avoiding others

Physical symptoms of stress

- Depression
- Anxiety
- Aches, pains, tense muscles
- Chest pain and rapid heartbeat
- Insomnia
- Frequent viral infections
- Low energy
- Lack of focus
- Headaches
- Upset stomach, including diarrhoea, constipation, nausea
- Nervousness and shaking
- Cold or sweaty hands and feet
- Excess sweating
- Dry mouth and difficulty swallowing
- Clenched jaw and grinding teeth

According to Centre for Disease Control and Prevention research, people who experience chronic stress are more prone to heart attacks, kidney disease, cancer, obesity and diabetes. They can suffer from sleep problems, digestive problems, fertility problems, urinary problems, depression, anxiety and a challenged immune system, making them more prone to viral infections such as flu or the common cold.

75-90% of all doctor's visits are for stress-related ailments and complaints. (Huffington Post). Stress can play a part in problems such as headaches, high blood pressure, heart problems, diabetes, skin conditions, asthma, arthritis, depression and anxiety.

Although as yet there is no strong evidence that stress directly affects cancer outcomes, some data suggests that patients can develop a sense of helplessness or hopelessness when stress becomes overwhelming. This response is associated with higher rates of death, although the mechanism for this process is unclear. It may be that people who feel helpless or hopeless do not seek treatment when they become ill, give up prematurely, or fail to adhere to potentially helpful therapy. They may engage in risky behaviours such as drug use. They are generally more neglectful of their health.

You can see why it is so vital for your health that you learn tools to improve the level of your executive functions.

In the UK and the USA more people than ever before are being prescribed anti-anxiety and anti-depressant medications. A major contributor to anxiety and depression is executive function deficit. I get frustrated that so many of my clients are on medication to manage their anxiety or depression.

These medications do have a place in patient treatment. The practitioners who are prescribing them, need to look at the root cause of the patient's problems, which is many cases is the patient's self-made crises due to their executive function deficit or ADHD. My clients regularly report feeling so much better when they integrate the tools to support their executive functions together with the ADHD meds. They feel so much better when they are on the right medications for their condition.

PART 3
YOUR ACTION TOOL KIT

THE FOUR TYPES OF FOCUS

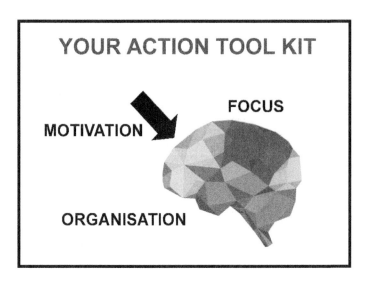

In this chapter you will understand how the executive functions of focus, motivation and organisation will help you to get things done. This is your very own action tool kit.

You may have heard that adults with ADHD can't pay attention. You may have heard that this is one of the main challenges associated with ADHD. This is not true. In reality, you focus on everything. You find it difficult to filter out the stimuli from your external environment and your internal environment, your thoughts, and to focus on one thing at a time.

There are four types of focusing powers. If you understand how to harness them in the right way, you can get much more done than other people who don't have ADHD.

The four types of focus are:

1. Hyperfocus
2. Hypofocus
3. Selective focus

4. Hovering focus

It is commonly thought that if you can focus for very long and intense periods of time then you can't have ADHD. This is one of the greatest myths about ADHD. You have an imbalance of attention. If you have ADHD you have the ability to *hyperfocus* and *hypofocus*, (though not at the same time). The focus powers on both sides of the scale can be enormously productive if you know how to harness them correctly.

Your *hyperfocus* is often visible in your areas of passion. In these areas you can stay focused, and your focus will be sharper and more intense for longer periods of time than most people. You have the potential to get so much done. The world needs people like you to hyperfocus on certain tasks. The downside of the hyperfocus strength is the difficulty you may experience in transitioning to regular focus mode, on time…and independently.

Your *hypofocus* is usually related to boring tasks. Do you find yourself getting distracted and then forgetting to return to your current task, often for many hours? You probably have many unfinished projects and tasks lying around the house. This contributes to your external environmental chaos and your internal feelings of chaos. Colleagues or family members are most likely unhappy with your performance. For your life success you need to find a way to work out how to stay focused on boring and overwhelming tasks until completion, no matter what!

Your *hypofocus* skills are essential for life. There are many tasks in life that require you to have your focus on many tasks at once, for example emergency personnel in a crisis zone need to focus on many facets of the situation at one time. You can learn to use your hypofocus skills to stay attentive to several tasks simultaneously, such as working on a team project. You may need strategies to enable you to come back to regular focus mode afterwards, independently and on time.

Selective focus is your ability to stay focused on tasks

even when there are distractions around you. This is a vital skill for your life success that can be mastered. It can be done. *Hovering focus* gets activated when you need to get some work done that requires effort and is not that engaging. Your ADHD brain needs constant entertainment and engagement. When your brain senses that boredom is about to set in it scans the environment for more fun activities. This is why when you start to work on an important project, you find yourself surfing the internet or going on social media for hours, (procrastination).

You need to first keep your hovering focus occupied before you can start to hyperfocus. You do this by working in an environment where there is noise or movement. Many clients like to study in their local library, or café, where there is background noise. This helps with focus. Listening to music (no words) also helps to keep the hovering focus at bay. I was able to finish writing this book by working in a shared office space for a few hours a day. The buzz and the noise of having people around me helped me to focus on the more tedious and boring task of editing and proof reading.

You hold the secret to your productive ADHD life. Become aware of your pattern of focus. Many people with ADHD relate that they can hyperfocus best at certain times of the day. Use your strengths wisely.

Your focus varies at different times of the day, week and even year. Start to observe yourself and see if you can detect a pattern. Then match your task to the appropriate level of focus.

One client noticed that she had peak performance in the months of May to July. She was super energised and was churning out projects. Her performance dipped dramatically during the months of November to February. During those months she was unmotivated, unfocused and quite depressed. SAD, Seasonal Affective Disorder, a condition that affects mood, energy and motivation is more common amongst those with ADHD. This is very common in women, especially in their mid 40s. More research is needed in this area.

Moira was a deeply frustrated mother of two young children. She was a talented florist. She sold flowers at certain busy times of the year to her community from her front room. She loved what she did. She really wanted to expand her business and rent a shopfront. She was frustrated with her inability to balance her work and home life. During the times when she ran her small business, she was up till 3am, in hyperfocus mode, working on her floral orders, and sleeping in till late in the morning, neglecting her household duties and her children.

Her husband was very unhappy about this. He saw how talented she was, how much potential her business had, however he was not prepared to put up with the huge mess at home, and the chaos in his children's lives while she was active in her business.

Through so many failed attempts, Moira started to believe that she could only be successful in one area, either be a stay-at-home mother or run a business. I showed her how she could actually do both successfully. Moira worked had for 6 months learning the ropes, and understanding how to harness her focus powers to work for her, not against her. She has recently rented a shopfront on her local high street. She has proven to herself that she can run her home smoothly and run her business successfully. Her self-esteem and self-confidence soared.

My clients have experienced the benefits of exercising after a session of intense hyperfocus to help them transition back into regular focus mode and maintain equilibrium and productivity.

Amy was behind with her assignment deadline. Her mentor gave her an extra 3 months to complete her work. She was having panic attacks and was on medication to manage her anxiety. Amy learnt to recognise her different focus strengths. She noted her optimum energy and focus levels, and learnt how to channel them to serve her goals. She learnt to pace herself and take frequent short breaks to exercise.

She found that it worked for her to get up at five am and do two hours of intense focused work. She took a quick break every half hour or so to run up and down the stairs or do some stretching. Then she gave her brain a break and did two hours of hypofocused work after that such as household chores and preparing for the day. Then she knew her brain could focus on another 1.5 hours of intense work. At around eleven am she felt her focus waning and started to feel restless. She went to the gym for a strenuous workout.

She understood how to change her work environment to give her brain a buzz and combat that feeling of boredom.

Amy made sure to spend some time in the middle of the day working on a totally different topic to give her brain the chance to 'switch off'. She continued with her intensely focused work for two hours later in the afternoon. Then she gave her brain a break until the evening, when she limited her work to two hours. Amy understood how to manage easier assignments in the evening when her teenagers were around using her selective focused mode.

Through pacing herself her anxiety lessened. She was able to function well again. She managed to complete her assignment on time with far less stress, and improved self-confidence.

Rachel was a client who wanted assistance with organising her house. She chose to start with her kitchen. After a couple of sessions, she got bored and wanted to start on the garage, before finishing the kitchen. We discussed the hypofocus idea and I asked Rachel how she could use this to help her complete the kitchen organisation first. She came up with the idea of shifting focus from one part of the kitchen to the other. When she completed one cupboard, she chose another one in a different part of the room but staying within the confines of those four walls. By sprinting from one part of the room to another she kept her brain engaged and buzzing. She managed to maintain focus to complete organising her kitchen.

During Ellen's first phone coaching session she set two intense goals for herself. She wanted to get to work on time, (her dream goal was to get into work 30 minutes early every day). Ellen was deeply ashamed that no matter how hard she tried, she rushed into work, in a mad tizzy at the last minute, often embarrassingly late, looking dishevelled and feeling all over the place and unfocused. She had run out of excuses a long time ago. She was fed up and ashamed. She desperately wanted to banish her late coming, but didn't know how to go about it. Her second goal was to get her house organised. She hadn't invited friends over in months. One day a friend popped in with ten minutes notice. She realised in horror that her friend was about to discover her darkest secret. She got into high gear. In ten minutes, she managed to tidy her home in a way that she hadn't done in over a year. When her friend left she realised it was time to stop covering up her intense shame, and get help.

During our phone session her husband James came on the line. He wasn't interested in Ellen's lofty goals. He just wanted her to close the kitchen cupboard doors after her, and put things away once they had been used. He was fed up with stuff lying about on the counters for days.

Ellen felt cheated and frustrated, as she wanted to focus on the big goals, but James was insistent that he wanted to see change in this area first before she tackled her other goals. I explained to Ellen that by simply working on one area, she would see improvement in other areas. I showed her how the difficulty that she had in closing cupboard doors and putting things away was directly related to her time management and organisational challenges.

I spent two sessions with James and Ellen just discussing the science behind her challenge with closing doors. Strategies only work when one understands the science that underpins them. The knowledge she gained empowered her, and helped her to realise that her challenges were not her fault. She was not a failure or a slob, she just had some skills that she needed to work on, that's all. Ellen started by focusing on closing kitchen cupboard doors only from 8:00 am till 9:00 am. She really wanted to spend more time working through her challenges, but I gently reminded her that long-term growth happens at a slow and steady pace.

Ellen set an alarm clock at 8:00 am to remind her to start closing the kitchen cupboard doors and put things away after use. She set a large timer on the kitchen table to keep her focused. She also got her family members to kindly encourage her. Ellen's progress was maddeningly slow.

This small goal of closing the kitchen cupboard doors and putting things away straight after use took Ellen many months of work before she saw improvement. Little by little, her daily actions increased her self-awareness. She became aware of her poor working memory in action, and how it had a direct impact on her mood. She also started to notice how her focus rapidly shifted from one task to the other, often sabotaging her best efforts for success. At first Ellen felt increasingly frustrated, as putting things away after use actually slowed her down. I supported her through this. After a couple of months, she saw a rise in her productivity levels between 8:00 and 9:00 am. She was confused about this. I explained that creating the habit of finishing a task, putting away the item after use and closing the cupboard door actually helped her become more efficient.

Ellen was fascinated that such a seemingly small goal had created such a huge impact on her productivity. She felt more energised than she had in years. She started getting to work earlier. She felt more motivation to get her housework done. She felt ready to seriously tackle the clutter in her garage. Ellen related that she felt more aligned with her values. She didn't need to excuse her failings to others. She accepted herself more, which made her feel more focused and peaceful.

Ellen took responsibility for her challenges, and focused on very small goals, with remarkable results.

MOTIVATION

Motivation, another executive function skill goes hand in hand with procrastination.

- Can you stay focused on your work without wandering off and forgetting to come back to finish it?
- Can you complete tasks that are boring, just as easily as jobs that are interesting, and complete them on time?
- When you start a project are you super motivated, but as you progress your enthusiasm fizzles out?
- Is your life plagued with incompletions? Are your incompletions holding you back from success?
- Do you have the ability to get to the finish line when the project inspires you?

Motivation means sticking to a project till the bitter (sweet) end. If you don't finish the task to the very last detail, it is as if you haven't started it (actually it is far worse!).

No one likes to be bored. It is an unpleasant emotional experience. Your ADHD brain is hard-wired for stimulation. You only feel alive when engaged in fun and exciting activities.

Dopamine is the chemical in your brain that is responsible for motivation. If you are an adult with ADHD your dopamine levels will not be working at their optimum levels. When you are bored dopamine levels dip drastically. When an activity is interesting, dopamine levels in the reward centre of your brain increase in response to the expectation of a reward. This then releases the energy you need to continue pursuing your activities. When your activity is boring, the reward centre in your brain does not get fired up. Without this good feeling that you get from the release of dopamine you will find it *impossible* to pursue your boring activity. Clients report that when they need to carry out a tedious or boring activity, they feel an internal block stopping them.

Now do you understand why following through on boring tasks is at best painful, and at worst, impossible to do, and feels like a living death.

OPEN THE DOOR TO YOUR INNER MOTIVATION

Your ADHD motivation is activated by how interesting the task is, not by how important the task is. Boring tasks are almost impossible to do. Many of my clients relate feeling an internal block when they need to get boring tasks done. They related that they feel an internal block that is stopping them from starting and getting the task done.

When your ADHD brain senses that the next task will be boring it wants to escape from the situation *right now!* Your focus starts to hover. Your brain scans the area for distraction and stimulation. If your brain doesn't find the what it wants you will likely start to engage in mind-numbing activities. You may turn to surfing the web, spending time on social media, or other activities that impact you and those around you in a negative way.

Learn to be pro-active, in other words, self-aware. If you sense yourself getting pulled to distraction, provide your hovering attention with a focus. Try using white noise or music (no words) to keep your brain buzzing. Doodle, or take notes. Try to incorporate movement while you work.

How does boredom feel like? When you become more aware how boredom feels inside your body you will be on the way to solving your challenge. You may feel frustrated or restless; you may lash out at others. Do you ever feel as though you are crawling out of your skin?

Aston had a lot of Skype meetings with his boss. To help him focus he would take off his shoes and roll the soles of his feet over a spikey ball. This sensation gave his hovering brain just the right amount of distraction, enabling him to give his full attention to the meeting.

When you become aware of your boredom, don't resist it. Welcome it and learn how to treat it. Are you hungry, stressed or sleep deprived? These are all contributing factors.

Sandwich boring activities between stimulating ones. A few minutes of intense exercise will raise the dopamine levels in your brain and energise you to continue with your tedious task.

The ironing was piled sky high in on Debora's couch. She HATED ironing and was at her wits end. Debora was on a tight budget and sending out her ironing to be done by someone else was not an option. She thought hard and found a solution. Once a week she would call a lonely great aunt whose conversation skills were less than stellar. It was not always easy to listen to her great aunt, and she found it really difficult to focus on the conversation. By keeping her brain busy with the repetitive actions of ironing, she started to be able to tune in and enjoy the weekly phone calls. Debora couldn't believe the results. After a few weeks she managed to get to the bottom of the ironing pile. Her ironing is now a weekly ritual that she ties in with the phone call.

Race against yourself. Set the timer and see how quickly you can complete the boring task. By moving fast, your actions arouse the reward centre in your brain, helping you feel stimulated and motivated.

Build up your resistance to discomfort. Little by little learn to tolerate boredom. Life is full of boring tasks. If you can succeed in turning those horribly boring tasks into interesting ones you have found your secret to task completion.

Stretching for a few minutes during a tedious activity is a great way to improve your focus and concentration.

John hosted a weekly get-together with his family. It was his responsibility to cook and prepare for this event. He hated cooking and found it terribly boring. He was fed up with his inability to plan and manage the preparations on time. The cooking felt like a heavy weight the entire week, and he was always late. John started to race against himself, and to prepare a fun activity with a friend straight after the cooking activity. This really got him motivated to start his cooking on time and stay focused.

Jason needed to complete his studies. He found it very difficult to focus at home in his room. His hovering brain craved the noise and energy of other people to help him concentrate. He tried studying in the library. The background noise kept his brain occupied but it was hard to get the right balance as sometimes the library was too noisy! Jason researched his area for a range of coffee shops and public places that he could use when needed. The variety of venues he frequented kept his brain buzzing and focused.

ORGANISATION

Organisation is another executive function skill. The disorganised state of your environment directly impacts your mental clarity and focus and vice versa. It is a never-ending cycle. You may be suffering from layers upon layers of disorganisation.

There are 3 types of organisation:

1. Home organisation
2. Mental organisation
3. Financial organisation

They are all linked together in your brain's executive functions. If you have a challenge in one area, you will likely have a challenge in other areas of organisation.

HOME ORGANISATION

This means that your belongings have a home, and their homes resonate with your lifestyle and your personality. Your belongings do not float around your home. You possess no clutter. You can find any item in your home, even an item that you haven't looked at in years, in under 3 minutes.

You probably organise and look after many people in your life. You could be really good at organising other people's belongings, but with your own stuff you may get totally overwhelmed. When you organise someone else's belongings, you don't get emotionally involved. When you need to sort your own stuff, your emotions play a vital role in sabotaging your success. When you experience negative emotions, you get overwhelmed and shut down. Do you have layers upon layers of stuff and papers that need organising?

Being organised means that your electrical equipment is in order. You don't own duplicates of the same items. You do not have tangles of random black wires lurking behind closed cupboard doors. When you are disorganised you feel dizzy and unfocused. This directly impacts your thoughts, emotions and actions.

MENTAL ORGANISATION

Your thoughts follow a logical sequence. You are able to write your thoughts down on paper in a clear, coherent fashion. You are able to verbalise your thoughts in a logical manner, without rambling on. During conversation you express yourself simply and eloquently. You don't waffle on and take absolutely ages to express a thought.

FINANCIAL ORGANISATION

Being organised means that your finances are in order and your financial papers are in order! You don't accumulate debt. If you *are* in debt you have a repayment plan in place. You keep to your budget, and save. Most importantly you know how you have spent your money. You can also keep track of the little things in life such as your keys and phone.

> Rinda had to get herself and her children up and ready to leave the house by 8:00 am every day. She felt completely frazzled. She needed a quick fix solution to help her get back on track. She made one small change. She took on the task of looking after her own needs before her family in the morning. Initially she was sceptical about it but decided to try it out anyway. She made sure to get herself dressed right away, did some stretches, and drank a cup of coffee before waking the children.
>
> By implementing these small changes consistently her mornings became calm and she was more in control. Her critical internal dialogue quietened down.

Mandy embarrassingly admitted that she kept losing her car keys. She even left them in her car door, sticking out of the keyhole on a number of occasions. She decided to tie a string through them and wear them around her neck. She wore it under her clothes so it was hidden. This method worked.

Agatha was 65 years old. She wanted to complete her thesis. She found it excruciatingly difficult to get through the necessary work. She had been given two extended deadlines, but she didn't need this. Agatha needed tools. She found it challenging to organise her work space, to ask for help, and to articulate her thoughts verbally and on paper. Her difficulty following instructions and in organising her thoughts stopped her from achieving her goal. Agatha learned how to break down her thoughts on paper, and how to keep to the relevant topic. She created a permanent work station. This grounded her and helped her brain focus. It was a painful and equally rewarding journey. She managed to reach the finish line, with two extended deadlines...

PART 4
YOUR PRODUCTIVITY TOOL KIT

FLEXIBLE THINKING

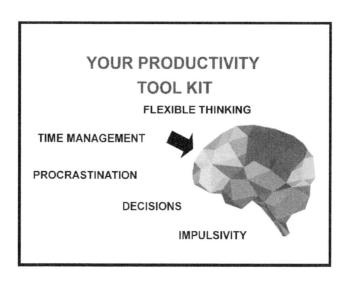

If you want to get more done in less time and with less effort, learn skills to improve the functioning of the above traits. They form the basis of your productivity tool kit.

Flexible thinking is one of the most important executive function skills you can acquire. According to Dr. Barkley (2013), one strength that many people with ADHD have is flexible thinking, the ability to come up with creative, out-of-the-box solutions to problems.

Flexible thinking can be broken down into six key areas.

1. Transitions – How easily can you adapt to new situations and transition from onetime frame/life stage to another?
2. Overwhelm – Can you independently break down complex tasks into bite size chunks?
3. Theory of mind – Are you able to see another person's viewpoint?

4. Problem solving – What are your problem-solving skills like? Can you see new and exciting possibilities where others see a brick wall?
5. Perfectionism – Do you view life in black and white or do you see lots of shades of grey?
6. Boundaries – Are you attentive to and mindful of boundaries?

All these skills can be learned.

TRANSITIONS

Life is synonymous with change. Day turns to night, seasons change, life moves on, friends move away, you get older. You need to use flexible thinking to adapt to those inevitable changes.

On one side of the scale you need change to keep you stimulated. On the other side, change is scary. How well you balance these two opposing forces will directly affect your success in life.

My clients are often creative free birds. They want freedom and creativity and resist routines. They think that routines and systems will tie them down. So we compromise. We set up routines for the key areas and leave out the rest. When your belongings have a home, when you have systems related to morning and evening routines, you will find it so much easier to transition from one setting to another, and one time frame to another. Systems actually liberate you.

OVERWHELM

Being overwhelmed is an offshoot of inflexible thinking. Here is the secret to facing it successfully. Challenge yourself to break down huge tasks into smaller bite-size ones. Then complete them one by one until you are done. The secret is to finish your tasks. Tie up those tedious, and boring lose ends.

Sarah's son Ron would leave a trail of mess wherever he went. When asked to tidy up, Ron would quickly get frustrated - often to the point of violent temper - and would often leave the job unfinished.

Sarah was fed up and wanted Ron to change. Through coaching she understood that he was not lazy or creating messes on purpose. She realised that he simply did not know how to break down the task of tidying up after himself. Sarah learned tools to teach him how to think flexibly and break down tasks into doable components.

Ron liked to make pizza for himself in their small grill oven. Sarah realised how many steps this task required, and praised Ron for accomplishing this by himself. After he had eaten she gently asked him to count how many items had been taken out of their places and now needed to be put away. He looked around and with her help, counted thirteen items.

Sarah asked Ron to put away the items. Ron couldn't remember where all the items belonged, so Sarah asked him to problem solve and guess which cupboard they lived in. He was able to do this with seven items. She helped him with the other six items by encouraging him to make educated guesses. With enough practise he will soon be able to do this independently without prompts.

THEORY OF MIND

If you want to get along with others you will need to develop your capacity for empathy. This is closely connected with flexible thinking.

When you are upset with someone, how easily can you understand their point of view? How easily do you understand their perspective on the situation? It is helpful talk this over with a friend. Sit in two chairs and role play the story. Then swap seats and act out the other person's viewpoint. When you repeat this often enough you will realise that there are many different ways to interpret an event. Life is not black and white. Life is endless shades of grey.

If you find yourself repeatedly getting upset with others, this may be a sign of emotional dysregulation. You find it challenging to regulate your feelings.

PROBLEM SOLVING

Creative people don't see problems, they see possibilities. When you are faced with a problem that looks like a wall, do you climb up a ladder or dig a tunnel? There is always a solution if you are creative enough to find one. You may be great at finding solutions for others but you may have a hard time finding those same solutions for yourself. Your emotions may be getting in the way. It is vital that you create a calm environment for yourself. This will have a huge impact on your ability to problem solve.

PERFECTIONISM

Do you torment yourself until you find the perfect solution? This world, the people in it and yourself, are imperfect. The perfect solution doesn't exist. Striving for excellence is far more realistic. If you do this then you will get more done in your life.

Eric, a trainee psychiatrist, felt deeply ashamed and guilty. Since the last session he hadn't completed his homework, which was finishing a presentation for a forthcoming convention. He felt under too much pressure to create the perfect presentation. Eric had managed to complete many other tasks that were equally important including another presentation for a different speech. Eric had also completed a load of dictations for his secretary, had updated a number of client portfolios, and had made great strides in his training. Eric realised that his feelings of failure due to not completing one of his tasks were caused by perfectionism, which was causing him great stress. He understood that for optimum productivity he needed to focus on what he was doing right. He suffered from anxiety, and realised that a large part was caused by his perfectionism, which was killing his satisfaction and joy of life.

We identified the potential difficulties that were stopping Eric from completing his presentation. He needed to do more research on the topic, as well as hash through his presentation ideas with a colleague - goals which he set for the following session. By understanding what was preventing him from reaching his goal and taking small, manageable steps, he managed to get the presentation completed on time.

Most importantly, Eric learned to replace his intense lifelong feelings of shame and guilt with self-acceptance and self-love.

BOUNDARIES

Being attentive to boundaries is another sub-skill related to flexible thinking. When you are asked to help someone are you attentive to your own boundaries? Do you find yourself adapting your life to meet your friend's needs when it doesn't always serve you well? Do you get easily taken advantage of? You just need to learn some skills to help you set personal boundaries and keep you safe. Saying 'yes' isn't always the correct choice. You might be helping others more than you should.

Remember when you say 'yes' to someone else you are often saying 'no' to yourself. Maintaining healthy boundaries is a delicate balance.

TIME MANAGEMENT

Your brain uses the same skills for time management, money management, possession management and paper management. When you work on only one of these areas, you will see a natural improvement in the other areas.

Rushing from one ADHD self-made crisis to the next is not an efficient way to live your life. If you are not managing your time well, you feel overwhelmed, and you believe that there is not enough time in the day to get your tasks done.

There are two ways you experience time: *flowing focus* or *fixed focus*. You can slip in and out of different focus states depending upon your external circumstances. Recognise your default time brain and take steps to support yourself.

FLOWING FOCUS BRAIN

If you have a flowing focus brain you see time as a concrete concept. You see the future coming towards you, and you plan accordingly. You are on time for appointments. You are the one in the family that keeps everything running smoothly. You exercise and take care of yourself. You are able to break down tasks into small chunks, and work at a steady pace towards your goals. You can independently tap into your inner motivation to get jobs done, especially boring tasks.

Do you have this flowing focus strength in all areas? Are you time-organised at work and at home?

FIXED FOCUS BRAIN

Everyone has a bit of the fixed focus brain. Here are some of its features.

You experience your life via intense emotions, both positive and negative. Your 'fight, flight and freeze' mechanism is on high alert, and gets easily aroused, making it hard to focus on tasks. You are likely to dwell on the negative emotional aspects of events. This can stop you from being as productive as you would like to be. You may distract yourself or escape from responsibilities, with negative repercussions.

It is not easy living with a fixed focus brain. Self-awareness and getting support are the critical steps needed to access a flowing focus brain.

Support your brain with easy to implement time tools. Focus on one small area of improvement, consistently for three months, and you will see a dramatic improvement in your life success.

PROCRASTINATION

- Do you have piles of projects started and not completed?

- Do you push off starting projects until the very last moment?

- Do you then get energised and pull an all-nighter (or a big chunk of it?)

When you learn how to overcome your procrastination you will improve your productivity. Understand that true fulfilment and satisfaction does not come from completing easy work. It comes from pushing through a difficult task to the best of your abilities. The satisfaction you experience upon completion is its own reward. So how do you start tasks on time and complete them way before the deadline?

There are four reasons why procrastination may be plaguing your life.

1. Perfectionism
2. Overwhelm
3. Confusion
4. Boredom

Your tasks in life will often be tedious and overwhelming. You may be tempted to shift focus to another task and return to your current job later. This is a trap! If you leave your current project unfinished you will probably never come back to complete the task.

PROCRASTINATION – BUSTER TOOLS

When you become aware of your thoughts and beliefs you are

on the way to change. It is all about self-awareness.

Do the following ideas resonate with you?

- "I must have the perfect plan. If I can't do the job perfectly, then I won't do it at all." Fear of failure and a high standard of perfection can paralyze you, and you may get lost in planning to perfection. This is incredibly frustrating as perfection does not exist.
- Do you become so excited about an idea or concept and let everyone else know how great it is? Do you spend all your energy promoting the idea rather than carrying it out?
- "When I've worked out all the pieces of the puzzle and all the people, then I will do what I need to do to get the job done." Are you waiting to see the whole picture before you can start?
- Do you make others believe you have been successful in similar types of projects before, but you are only talking to feel better?
- Do you put off a project until the deadline is looming, and the adrenaline rush kicks in?
- Do you feel so overwhelmed by what you want to do that the idea of failing blurs your vision and prevents you from taking the first steps?
- Do you tell yourself that you must finish your task, thereby putting pressure on yourself, and emotional shut down follows very soon after.

If you are confused, don't be ashamed to ask for help. Don't give up until your problem is clarified. It is the clever people that ask for help.

Do you find yourself aiming for very high (read unrealistic) standards? Just aim for the 'good enough' level. Just start!

Create a 'body double'. Find a friend to keep you

company when you need to tackle a tedious, complicated task. Having another person around gives your brain a buzz and helps you to keep focused.

Don't aim to finish as task, aim to start it. The hardest part is starting. Once you have started the task, it is easier to move along towards your end goal.

If you are feeling overwhelmed, simply break down the mammoth task into small, bite size chunks. Only focus on getting the very next step done. This is a skill that can be learned.

Emily was able to get started on her holiday cooking marathon on time through breaking down the various stages of her cooking process. The night before she laid out the ingredients on the counter. In the morning it was much easier to start on her to-do list because she had already 'started' the night before.

Julie, an accountant, had ADHD. Her brain would pull her attention all over the place. She could count on one hand how many projects she had actually completed in her life. She was unhappy with this situation. At one point her boss threatened to sack her.

Julie decided to learn strategies to help herself. When she needed to focus on a tedious project, she allowed herself to jump from one topic to another within that project until she successfully completed it. She started to work part time from home to create variety in her week. She learnt how to keep her buzzing mind on task and engaged.

Ray was 18 years old. All through his school and college studies Ray had always hated studying. He had never completed an assignment on time or to the required level.

Ray approached me because he had failed his grades at college and wanted help. He didn't want to work as a sales boy his entire life, and realised that with a better education he would be more likely to get a better job.

Ray had many strengths, which we spent time enumerating. He was very creative. He was also a visual thinker. He needed to verbalise his thoughts in order to really understand the subject matter. I showed him how to draw out the assignment on a large paper. He then drew the components to the assignment using icons, adding colour to his drawing.

He had always thought of himself as someone who was lazy and who hated studying. Now he understood that he simply needed to adapt the study methods and learning material to suit his personal way of learning. I showed him how to break down his work assignments into small doable chunks. By doing this he started to enjoy studying, something he had not achieved for his entire life.

We discussed how to improve his nutrition, and his sleep. Ray became more self-aware, tuning into his optimum energy levels and harnessing them to improve his studies.

Ray's assignment was due in a month's time. He printed out the next month's calendar, and drew each assignment component onto the next month.

He worked backwards, starting from the day before the assignment was due. He then assigned a time frame when each component needed to be completed. Ray gave himself plenty of time to complete each part.

Over the next month I stayed in touch with Ray via email, giving him the necessary support to stay on task and complete the assignment. After handing in the assignment on time, he sent me the following email:

"This has been the first time in my life that I have actually enjoyed studying for an exam! I have stayed on target throughout the study period. Most importantly I did not lose any sleep over this! I now feel energised and motivated to continue moving forward. I have the confidence that I possess and the tools to help me reach my goals."

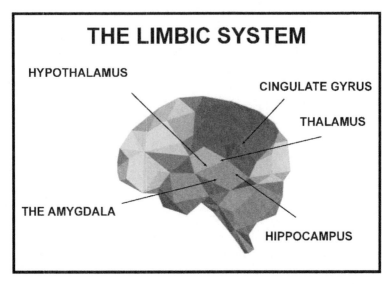

THE LIMBIC SYSTEM

HYPOTHALAMUS

CINGULATE GYRUS

THALAMUS

THE AMYGDALA

HIPPOCAMPUS

You have read about your limbic system earlier in the book. Your limbic system comprises:

1. Thalamus
2. Hypothalamus
3. Cingulate gyrus
4. Bilateral amygdala
5. Hippocampus

It is your security guard, monitoring your surroundings for potential danger and threats. If it perceives any form of danger it will kick into high alert.

Your limbic system cannot differentiate between different types of fear. When you feel anxiety over an upcoming project, your limbic system works against you; you will either become angry, distract yourself, or shut down.

When your limbic system is working at full blast, essentially to protect you, it hijacks your brain. All of your executive functions shut down. You are unable to get your work done or think rationally. You must first calm down (this may take some time) and only then focus on the internal processes.

When you are faced with an overdue deadline that is sending you into panic mode, or a new idea or project that you would love to start, but you are feeling really anxious about, you have just five seconds to get started before the negative feeling totally overtakes your rational mind, and your limbic system starts to work against you. If you have a project deadline that is giving you grief, get up and do one small related task. If you have an ingenious idea, get up straight away and make one small contribution towards that idea, no matter how afraid you may feel. It will now be much easier to follow that trajectory. In this way you will have started, and once you have started your limbic system calms down.

DECISIONS – TOO MANY POSSIBILITIES

The art of deciding with focus and ease, and knowing how to prioritise your time is an executive function skill.

- Do you torment yourself and your family members when you need to make a decision?
- Does it take you time to process information? Do you sense that you work at a different pace to others?
- When you have made a decision, do you torment yourself endlessly because you simply can't remember the steps that you took to make that decision?
- Have you lost out on significant life opportunities because you just couldn't decide?
- Are you looking for the perfect solution?
- When you need to make a decision, do you get exhausted easily?

You need to make decisions thousands of times a day. Some of those decisions are important, some are not. This morning you decided whether to get out of bed or to sleep in. You decided what to wear, and what to eat for breakfast. You decided to answer that urgent text, rather than leave it for later.

Decisions are tough. The decision-making process puts a huge strain on your executive functions. You need to think on your feet in a split second. As you progress through the day your brain gets tired, and it gets harder to decide quickly and easily. Your emotions often prevent you from deciding with ease. The torment taxes your brain, tiring you further.

If you have problems with decision-making please understand that it may be difficult for your brain to recognise and prioritise what is important to you and what you can filter out.

FIVE DECISION-MAKING TIPS

1. Apply the 'good enough' solution
2. Narrow your possibilities
3. Support your working memory
4. Pay attention to one thing at a time
5. Trust your instinct

THE 'GOOD ENOUGH' SOLUTION

Have you ever experienced decision paralysis? This feeling of paralyzed overwhelm occurs when you want the entire cake. Realistic decision makers understand that they may only be able to eat one piece of the cake, and this is good enough. They understand that they may have to negotiate their ideal plan, and settle for an outcome that is vastly different from their original plan. Great decision makers understand this and decide quickly.

Common paralysing thought patterns are:

"Maybe I should…" and you continue thinking of alternatives.

"But what if…?" And you think of all the possible consequences of your decision.

"I want to wait a bit longer before deciding to make sure that I don't make a mistake."

Are you waiting for that perfect time? The perfect time is right now. The past is over, the future is not yet here. The longer you waver in no man's land of indecisiveness, the more time you waste your present life. Your fear of failure is real. If you want to achieve your goals in life you will need to face your fears, challenge them and work through them. Your fears will not go away, if you don't face them, they will just get bigger.

When you need to decide on a course of action, there is no way in the world that you can have *all* options available to you. There will *always* be some piece of information that is missing. You need to be brave and jump in and decide with the knowledge that you have access to right now.

If you are trying to find the perfect answer, understand that you are searching for that elusive pot of gold at the end of the rainbow. *It does not exist.* Every decision that you will ever make closes another door of possibility.

Every time you decide you should expect to lose out in some way. Such is life. Realise that you have formed your decision with the best tools and knowledge available to you. Then move on.

If you think that you will simply refrain from making a decision, and let nature take its course, please understand that you are choosing the route of the losers in life.

June was a science teacher in a local high school. She was fed up with her job, having been in the same place for 10 years. Over the last two years she had tried really hard to bring creativity and innovation to her department but the head teacher showed little interest in supporting her in any way. From one day to the next, June decided to leave and move on with her life.

The day after her decision she found out a piece of information that, had she known about it, she might have stayed.

She still remained confident about her decision as she knew that at the time of her decision, she had decided with the best tools available to her knowledge at the time. Five years down the line she is delighted with her current position

NARROW YOUR POSSIBILITIES - LESS REALLY IS MORE!

- Do you get overwhelmed with the myriad details and endless possibilities when making a decision?
- Do you get headaches or suffer physical pain when you need to make major decisions?

Narrow your options. Less really is more. Some people are great at seeing the details of an idea, and some are better at seeing the big picture. For great decision-making you will need to be able to view both simultaneously. This will only be achievable when you narrow your options.

Decide on a time frame and a deadline when you will make your decision.

Erica found shopping an absolute nightmare. So many choices! So many possibilities! When she entered shops, she often became disoriented and overwhelmed. She usually left the shop empty handed, and came home with a splitting headache. She hadn't bought anything new in years. Her wardrobe consisted of a few lonely items, all mismatched. Her self-image plummeted.

I taught Erica how to create a personalised capsule wardrobe. She narrowed the colours of her wardrobe to shades of grey, blue and pink. She decided to only patronise three favourite shops. She was amazed how easy her shopping experience became. She drastically reduced the time she spent shopping. Most importantly she replaced her dizziness and confusion with calm and clarity. Her cupboard is now full of stylish clothes that she can mix and match with ease. Most importantly she feels super confident, and as a result has made some wise forward-thinking business decisions.

SUPPORT YOUR WORKING MEMORY

Decision-making paralysis is a sign of a poor working memory.
Your decision overwhelm may simply be a sign of your working memory deficit. Your working memory is like a mental post-it note. If you have a poor working memory you will find it difficult to keep the many facets affecting your decision in the forefront of your mind.

In addition to this sometime after the decision has been made, you may regret and doubt yourself because *you can't remember the factors that helped you form that decision!* If your decision is proven to have been unwise you may blame yourself or others for your mistakes, getting twisted up in knots. If you can't remember the steps that you took to form a decision, and that decision has gone awry, others may blame you, and if you can't defend your decision you will look incompetent and foolish.

Support your working memory by offloading via a journal. Write the pros and cons of your decision. This will help you focus, and will serve as a written record for the future. If you start to doubt yourself you can always refer back to your journal for reference and peace of mind.

1. You may be a verbal processor. Hashing out your thoughts with a friend will probably be more helpful than putting your thoughts onto paper. Go through the various aspects of your decision process with a trusted friend to help you decide.

2. You may be a visual processor. Draw your thoughts on paper using simple icons. Use colour to help you focus.

3. The best way to improve your decision-making skills is to make more and more decisions! The more you push through your fears, and make decisions, the easier it becomes to face them bravely.

What happens to you when you face your fears? You become a more genuine person. People will be drawn to you as your inner spiritual light becomes apparent. Note that once you have come to a decision, barring exceptional circumstances, stick to that decision as it builds your character.

I worked with Alex for six months, organising her home. She chose to start with organising her kitchen as the clutter was getting in her way. Three sessions on, she regretted her decision. She really wanted to move on to the paperwork. She couldn't understand why she had decided to work on the kitchen first. The papers were driving her insane. I gently reminded her of her reasons why she decided to start with the kitchen. She looked at me in wonder. She could not recall those ideas. I acted as her external working memory.

PAY ATTENTION TO ONE THING AT A TIME

If you have ADHD you may believe that you can't pay attention. The real challenge for you and other adults with ADHD is that you pay attention to everything! You have a surplus of attention. You find it difficult to shift your focus to only one stimulus. Your attention is drawn, not only to the stimuli in your environment, but to the stimuli in your internal world, your thoughts.

With all your thoughts swirling around in your head, deciding which thoughts to pay attention to when making a decision, can be totally overwhelming. Since it can be so difficult to focus your attention on one thought at a time, you may avoid thinking about your decision, or impulsively make a decision, without thinking it through enough, or continue being immersed in your inner world, and not do anything.

The antidote to this challenge is to take the time to slow down and gather your thoughts. You need to come out of your head, and become grounded in your body. Hash it out with a trusted friend, or write down your thoughts in a journal.

You may be avoiding deciding simply because you need to make a few pre-decisions before you make your final decision. This is totally normal. Just slow down and focus on each decision.

TRUST YOUR INSTINCT

If you have made many decisions in the past that you were not happy with, you may have lost trust in your ability to decide successfully. Gather all the information that you need to decide and listen to your inner voice, that is there, but may have been quietened due to you ignoring its message for so long. The more that you bravely decide with your instinct, the more you will become successful at decision-making.

One way to do this is to physically take yourself away from the situation.

- Go for a walk
- Sleep on it
- Wait for a certain time frame, a day or two, then commit to decide
- Do something totally unrelated to the decision.

In this way you allow your subconscious brain to process the information. You may be pleasantly surprised at the messages your inner voice, (your instinct) will give you.

IMPULSIVITY/SELF-CONTROL

Your level of self-control, or how well you can control your impulses, is another executive function skill. Your barometer of self-control determines how successful you will be in reaching your life goals. The more self-aware you become, the easier it will be to control impulses such as blurting, reacting, spending, eating and more.

Self-control has two parts:

- Self-control is the ability to do the boring, repetitive, but fundamental tasks that are an essential part of your life, even when you don't feel like it. Can you stick to those tasks even when new and exciting ideas and opportunities come your way?
- Self-control is the ability to say 'no' to yourself, even when you really don't want to, in order to match the standards of those around you.

Ask yourself the following questions:

- Are you able to stop yourself from blurting out inappropriate comments in social settings?
- Do you make a lot of impulsive purchases?
- Do you suffer from addictive behaviours such as eating?
- Do you have unusually strong willpower when the action speaks to your values?
- How good are you at living your life with firm, regular routines and habits?

Routine forms the basis for all your creative pursuits. Routine frees up your time and resources to pursue your creative side. When your daily tasks are organised, you will have more time, energy and focus to devote to the creative things that you love.

It took many years for Veronica to realise that she had an impulsive spending problem. When she was bored this became worse. She found it very difficult resisting the urge to buy something. Slowly she learned to say "no" to herself, even talking loudly to herself when out in public. She wasn't embarrassed to "make a fool of herself" because she knew too well the negative ramifications of her impulsive spending habits.

Ali was in her early twenties, with a diagnosis of ADHD. She had tried over 50 therapies and medications to help her, with little success. She understood that her many talents were useless unless contained in the vessel of executive functions.

Ali decided to go for coaching as a last-ditch effort. Her goals were to improve her productivity and get her life back on track.

Ali's 'normal' routine was to go to sleep at 3:00 am, and wake up at 1:00 pm. She wanted to start a job but knew that first, her unhealthy sleeping pattern needed to stop. She was aware that part of the problem was the evening WhatsApp group that she was part of.

During her second coaching session she impulsively called out, "That's enough!" She typed out a final message to her WhatsApp group on the spot and signed out forever. She set up a password system that only I had access to and blocked all her internet and social media after 11:00 pm. Ali was absolutely terrified but she knew that I was there to support her. It was now or never.

The first morning after the 'impulsive' change she related that she had gone to bed at 12.30 am, a huge improvement. Little by little over the coming months, with some bumps along the way, she got her life back on track.

PART 5
UNDERSTAND YOUR ADHD

ADHD FACTS – TRUE OR FALSE?

How well do you understand ADHD?

- **Myth No. 1 – ADD is a separate condition from ADHD.**
  ADHD and ADD are basically the same condition, except for the 'H' as in 'Hyperactivity'.

- **Myth No 2 – ADHD does not exist.**
  ADHD is a real biological disorder. ADHD can be detected in brain imaging scans. Major differences have been detected between the ADHD brain and the neurotypical brain. ADHD is transferred from parent to child. (Demontis, et al. 2017). ADHD is present worldwide and even in remote population groups. (Azevedo, 2010).

- **Myth No 3 – ADHD is a childhood condition that will eventually go away on its own.**
  ADHD was once commonly thought to only affect children. Current research has found that up to 65% of children with ADHD will have disabling symptoms into adulthood and throughout their lives (Cherkasova, et al. 2013).

- **Myth No 4 – If I simply ignore the problems created by ADHD they will eventually disappear.**
  The problems caused by ADHD *never* disappear. The challenges associated with unmanaged ADHD can be so all-consuming that even intelligent, successful adults with ADHD suffer from their symptoms, often leading to demoralising results (Cherkasova et al. 2013). ADHD is not a fatal condition. The problems that arise as a result of untreated ADHD can be fatal.

- **Myth No 5 – ADHD occurs on its own without a comorbid condition.**
  Up to 80% of those diagnosed with ADHD will have a second co-morbid condition (National Resource Centre on ADHD 2003).

- **Myth No 6 – The ADHD meds are poison. They should not be given to children or adults.**
  Unfortunately, ADHD medications have received bad coverage in the media. Much of the opposition stems from ignorance. They are powerful and need to be monitored carefully.

  Consider the following: If you or a family member has been diagnosed with ADHD you need to ask yourself, *"Living with your ADHD is hard. Do you deserve to have a more difficult life than other people just because you were born with ADHD?"*

- **Myth No 7 – If I give ADHD meds to my child, he/she will be cured.**
  Research has shown that ADHD medication helps with roughly a third of the symptoms (Barkley, 2010). The rest of the symptoms will require different forms of therapy to teach the person life skills (executive function skills).

- **Myth No 8 – I can't tell my family that I have ADHD because I am too embarrassed.**
  In the USA, great strides have been made in addressing ADHD and bringing it out into the open. In other places, such as the UK, the stigma associated with ADHD is still great, but change is happening little by little. Your ADHD is not your fault. You didn't cause your ADHD. You have nothing to hide.

- **Myth No 9 – My child has ADHD. If I'm firm with him, then he will surely behave.**

This is not true. The child with ADHD needs special parenting strategies. Trying to whip a child into shape will do great harm. Parenting a child with ADHD is undoubtedly challenging, but when carried out with the right tools and outlook, can be extremely rewarding.

- **Myth No 10 – At least my child only has ADHD. There are other mental health conditions that are much worse.**
  You are right. There may be other mental health conditions that are more serious. I have personally seen the far-reaching debilitating repercussions associated with unmanaged ADHD among my clients.

WHAT IS ADHD?

The term ADHD is short for Attention Deficit Hyperactive Disorder.

The term 'disorder' is misleading. Those with ADHD are not 'disordered', they are 'different' and have very special talents and gifts, and challenges. There is no such thing as a 'normal' brain. Every person is unique. We need to celebrate the unique strengths of each individual, and value the contribution that they can make to the world. When channelled in the right way, ADHD is a real strength.

A client summed it up very well. "ADHD is neither good nor bad. Your ADHD is a tool to be harnessed for positive or negative. It is up to you how you use your ADHD. You can either use it to mess up your life, or you can use it to transform your life."

If you have ADHD you will have executive function deficit. Understand that you can have executive function deficit without having ADHD.

ADHD is diagnosed after the age of six where the following is observed:

1. An increase in symptoms of inattention
2. An increase in hyperactivity
3. An increase in impulsivity

These behaviours must be present in two out of three situations; at school, in the clinic and at home.

ADHD is characterised by the inability to organise behaviour over time and prepare for the future. It is the inability to regulate emotions and gain self-control, to prioritise, make decisions and get tasks done in a timely fashion.

If you have ADHD you will experience challenges with your executive functions, including impulsivity, hyperactivity, attention deficit and distractibility. Inconsistency in performance lies at the heart of ADHD.

ADHD does not affect your intelligence levels.

Your creativity and inner resources far outweigh your ADHD deficits. You are probably highly intuitive, creative and resourceful. The world needs you and your unique strengths!

Your ADHD is separate from who you are and from your innate value as a person. No one can take your core value and inherent goodness away from you.

Knowledge and acceptance of your ADHD bring empowerment and growth.

ADHD is a biological condition, clearly recognizable in brain scans. There are five areas in the brain that are associated with the delayed development of ADHD.

ADHD is a genetic neurodevelopmental condition whereby some parts of the brain remain partially undeveloped, and are smaller in size than neuro-typical brains.

Your brain development impacts your behaviour. If ADHD is a developmental delay, your brain age (in the area of your ADHD deficits) may be far younger than that of your peers, commonly up to ten years or more behind. Conversely, in your areas of strength, your brain age may be more developed than that of your peers. You are living with a confusing mix of great strengths and deficits.

ADHD is one of the most treatable mental health conditions.

ADHD is genetic; if you or your child has ADHD *it is not your fault*. If you have a parent with ADHD, you are eight times more likely to have it. ADHD is present across all cultures (Azevedo, et al. 2010).

Studies have found that being born prematurely (before the 37th week of pregnancy), having a low birthweight, smoking, or alcohol or drug abuse during pregnancy may be risk factors for having ADHD (Harris, et al. 2013).

The difference between just having ADHD traits, which we all do, and getting diagnosed with ADHD is F.I.D. This stands for Frequency, Intensity and Duration. Dr. Barkley (2013) has conducted an in-depth study on this topic. His findings clearly indicate that those with ADHD have more significant impairments than those without ADHD. Here is a sample from his study comprising some ninety questions:

- Can't seem to persist at tasks that they find boring
  ADHD 96%; non-ADHD 13%
- Can't seem to get things done unless there is an immediate deadline
  ADHD 89%; non-ADHD 6%
- Trouble organising thoughts
  ADHD 80%; non-ADHD 4%
- Waste or mismanage time
  ADHD 86%; non-ADHD 5%
- Prone to daydreaming when they should be focusing on a task
  ADHD 96%; non-ADHD 3%

(Dr. Russell Barkley, "Taking Charge of Adult ADHD" page 271).

NATURE VERSUS NURTURE

The age old argument is ADHD caused by trauma or is it passed down in the genes?

ADHD is never caused by trauma. When the brain has been through trauma, it will exhibit ADHD symptoms until the trauma is processed. Trauma can also lead to the ADHD condition being activated. This only happens when the genetic element is already present.

Undiagnosed and unsupported ADHD can also lead to trauma, making the ADHD symptoms worse.

Environment can never cause ADHD. If it is in the genes, then the environment can activate or suppress it. Tobacco, stress, trauma, pregnancy, screen time, lack of play, can all activate the ADHD. If ADHD is in the genes it will most likely come out at some point during the lifespan. (www.adhdwise.co.uk)

THE THREE TYPES OF ADHD

ADHD is divided into three sub-types

- Inattentive type, (ADD)
- Hyperactive-impulsive type, (ADHD)
- Combination of the above two types, (ADHD combined)

In the following symptom breakdown, you will recognise the core executive function deficits that play a major role in your ADHD sub-type. Your symptoms will determine which type of ADHD you have. We all have a bit of ADHD in us. To be diagnosed with ADHD, symptoms must have an impact on your day-to-day life and be present across all settings. Symptoms can change over time, so the type of ADHD you have may change, too.

The 3 core criteria for an ADHD diagnosis are:

- Inattention: getting distracted, having poor concentration and organisational skills
- Impulsivity: interrupting, taking risks, struggling with self-control
- Physical hyperactivity: always on the go, never seeming to slow down, talking and fidgeting, difficulty staying on task, non-stop racing thoughts

PREDOMINANTLY INATTENTIVE ADHD (ADD)

In the UK this type of ADHD is called ADD, (without the H).

If you have this type of ADHD, you may experience more symptoms of inattention than those of impulsivity and hyperactivity. You may struggle with impulse control or hyperactivity at times. But these aren't the main characteristics of inattentive ADHD.

The person with ADHD typically:

- Has difficulty organising thoughts and learning new information
- Has problems with organising their belongings and papers
- Has a working memory deficit
- Misses details, misunderstands information more than others, and is easily distracted
- Gets bored quickly, and shifts focus often
- Has trouble focusing on a single task
- Moves slowly and appear as if they're daydreaming
- Processes information more slowly and less accurately than others
- Has trouble following directions
- Loses pencils, papers, or other items needed to complete a task
- Doesn't seem to listen

PREDOMINANTLY HYPERACTIVE-IMPULSIVE ADHD

This type of ADHD is characterised by symptoms of impulsivity and hyperactivity. People with this type can display signs of inattention, but it's not as marked as the other symptoms.

People who are impulsive or hyperactive often:

- Has trouble engaging in quiet activities
- Talk constantly
- Touch and play with objects, even when inappropriate to the task at hand
- Blurt out answers and inappropriate comments
- Squirm, fidget, or feel restless

- Have difficulty sitting still
- Are impatient
- Act out of turn and don't think about consequences of actions

COMBINATION ADHD (COMBINED ADHD)

If you have the combination type, it means that you have a combination of symptoms from both of the categories are exhibited.

Most people, with or without ADHD, experience some degree of inattentive or impulsive behaviour. But it's more severe in people with ADHD. The behaviour occurs more often and interferes with how you function at home, school, work, and in social situations.

Most children have combination type ADHD. The most common symptom in preschool-age children is hyperactivity.

Everyone is different, so it's common for two people to experience the same symptoms in different ways. For example, these behaviours are often different in boys and girls. Boys may be seen as more hyperactive, and girls may be quietly inattentive

IS ADHD A MODERN-DAY CONDITION?

If anyone tells you that ADHD is a figment of the modern imagination, show them this chapter.

ADHD has been around for a very long time. In *the Hippocratic Corpus, Volume IV* (450-350 BCE) there is a description of a condition that resembles an aspect of what we now know as ADHD.

The symptoms of inattention, hyperactivity, and impulsivity, all core traits of ADHD, have been recorded at various times over the last two hundred years. One of the very first descriptions of what might have been ADHD was by Scottish physician Sir Alexander Crichton in 1798. He wrote a book called 'Diseases of Attention', which brought to light symptoms of inattention in a group of school children, which at the time were labelled 'the fidgets'.

German physician Heinrich Hoffmann published an illustrated children's story titled *Struwwelpeter*, about 'Fidgety Phil' in 1845 who sounded like he probably displayed the hyperactive-impulsive symptoms of ADHD:

> *"Let me see if Philip can be a little gentleman; let me see if he is able to sit still for once at the table. Thus, Papa bade Phil behave; and Mamma looked very grave. But fidgety Phil, he won't sit still. He wriggles and giggles. And then, I declare, swings backwards and forwards, and tilts up his chair, just like any rocking horse. "Philip! I am getting cross!" See the naughty restless child growing still more rude and wild, till his chair falls over quite..."*

Hoffman wrote another book called *The Story of Johnny Head-In-Air*, which describes one possible symptom of ADD:

> *"It was always Johnny's-rule*
> *To be looking at the sky*
> *And the clouds that floated by;*

But what just before him lay,
In his way,
Johnny never thought about."

No mention was made of ADHD, but the symptoms match with those in the American Psychiatric Association's DSM-5, the current Diagnostic and Statistical Manual of Mental Disorders.

In 1902 Sir George Still was the first to publish his observations of a condition that looks like ADHD in a medical journal. He called it a 'defect of moral control' His findings were published in The Lancet. He was the first to note the unbalanced ratio between boys and girls affected (15 boys to 5 girls). His opinion was that one of the core qualities of this condition being self-gratification.

In 1932, German physicians Franz Kramer and Hans Pollnow described a condition that they called 'hyperkinetic disease of infancy', where the most striking symptom was a marked motor restlessness. The children they studied showed no perseverance in many activities, yet they were able to persevere for hours at activities in which they were especially interested. They came to call the disorder a 'hyperkinesis of childhood' because the signs of hyperactivity declined as the children grew up. They were the first ones to separate this from other disorders. Their description is similar to modern day ADHD.

In 1937 Dr. Charles Bradley discovered that stimulant drugs such as Benzedrine (an amphetamine compound) improved the behaviour of children who had been hospitalized with behavioural problems. He had been attempting to treat them for headaches caused by neurological examinations. Although the Benzedrine, an amphetamine compound, did not cure the headaches, he noticed that many children experienced significant improvements in behaviour and school performance after taking it. (Lange et al. 2010).

He started a trial of the medication with 30 children and

found that they performed better at school. Some children also experienced a decrease in motor activity and became more emotionally stable. He later found that the children who benefited the most from Benzedrine were those who had short attention spans, dyscalculia, mood instability, very high and very low moods, hyperactivity, impulsivity, and poor memory.

Being that Benzedrine is a stimulant, Dr. Bradley's discovery was revolutionary. His report had almost no influence on research for approximately 25 years. This was possibly due to the popularity of psychoanalysis as a treatment at the time.

From the early 1900s, right up until the early 1960s the medical world viewed brain damage to be the major cause of the hyperkinetic condition.

In the 1960s there was a shift in thought that led to 'minimal brain damage' moving into 'minimal brain dysfunction'.

By 1966 the three symptoms of impairment of control; attention, impulses, and motor functions were established as the central criteria for minimal brain dysfunction.

In 1968, the second edition of the Diagnostic and Statistical Manual of Mental Disorders (DSM-II) described Hyperkinetic Reaction of Childhood: 'The disorder is characterized by over- activity, restlessness, distractibility and short attention span, especially in young children; the behaviour usually diminishes by adolescence'.

In 1980, the American Psychiatric Association renamed the disorder 'Attention Deficit Disorder (ADD) (with or without hyperactivity)' (DSM-III). In this version, there were three separate lists of symptoms for inattention, impulsivity and hyperactivity.

Due to ongoing debate, the disorder was renamed 'Attention Deficit-Hyperactivity Disorder (ADHD)' in the 1987 revision of the third edition, and the symptom lists were combined. They also removed the subtype 'ADD without Hyperactivity' and put it in an 'undifferentiated ADD' category.

In the 1990s, professionals recognised that ADHD was a condition that did not disappear with age. It remained chronic and persistent into adulthood and throughout life. The DSM-III-R, in 1994, divided ADHD into three distinct subtypes: predominantly inattentive, predominantly hyperactive-impulsive and the two combined, and it added examples of workplace difficulties to demonstrate how symptoms presented in adulthood.

Around that time Dr. Alan Zametkin found reduced blood flow and lower metabolism of glucose in the frontal lobes of the brain, specifically the pre-frontal cortex, when those with ADHD were doing tasks that required thinking and focus. (Zametkin, et al. 1990).

In 2013, the DSM-IV removed the subtypes due to concern that they were confusing to diagnosticians.

More ongoing vital research is being carried out that will help shape the way that ADHD is viewed by the public and treated by mental health professionals.

ADHD MISNAMED

Until recently, medical professionals focused primarily on the attention span aspect of ADHD. Studies have revealed that the emotional dysfunction is far more common and disabling than the hyperactive and impulsive dysfunction of ADHD. Mental health professionals who specialise in diagnosing ADHD often overlook the most challenging symptom of ADHD; the emotional world of their patients. It is the inability to manage and successfully control emotions that lies at the heart of the condition. Anger management issues, overreacting without thinking things through, being super-sensitive to criticism, overwhelming negative thought patterns, depression, anxiety, overwhelm shutdown, crippling fear and worry are just some of the symptoms of the ADHD emotional dysfunction. Challenges in regulating the extreme positive emotions lie on the opposite side of the scale.

These emotional difficulties have a far greater impact than the attention difficulties. Emotional self-regulation affects every part of one's life including family life, work life and social life. You can forgive a friend for arriving late, or spacing out for a few minutes during a conversation. The same friend will not be so easily forgiven for lashing out at you or shouting at his boss, co-worker or spouse. Driving and criminal offences will not be overlooked due to ADHD either. A very high proportion of people in prison have ADHD.

When a client mentions that they may have ADHD, I am more concerned with their levels of emotional self-regulation than their focusing challenges.

ADHD treatment should focus primarily on becoming self-aware and learning how to recognise and control irregular and often overwhelming and stormy emotions.

WHAT IS HAPPENING INSIDE YOUR ADHD BRAIN?

Below is a diagram showing the main areas in the brain affected by ADHD

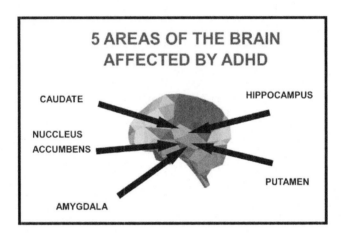

ADHD affects at least 5 different areas of the brain.

1. Amygdala
2. Caudate
3. Hippocampus
4. Putamen
5. Nucleus accumbens

In those with ADHD there are reduced amounts of the neurotransmitters dopamine and norepinephrine in the brain. Medications used to treat ADHD work by increasing the levels and availability of these chemicals in the brain.

The brain is divided into several areas, each with its own specific job. There is a thin, white outer layer called the **cerebral cortex**. This is where most of your thinking and learning takes place, and where memory is stored.

Under the cortex is a layer called the **subcortex**. The subcortex helps you stay alert and coordinates your brain's activities. It contains the **relay system**, which does many jobs. The relay system takes in information from your senses and redirects it to the correct department inside the cortex. It determines what to pay attention to, sending messages to 'turn on' other parts of your brain. This includes the "self-control" system. The centre for your emotions (anger, fear, happiness, or excitement) and the "reward centre" (an area that becomes active when something gives you pleasure or makes you happy) are also located here. This may explain why you can focus better when you are carrying out an activity that you enjoy, or one that you know you'll receive a reward for when you finish.

The brain is made up of billions of **neurons** – cells that work together although they do not touch each other. They are separated by a tiny space called a **synapse**. The neurons send messages to each other through chemical messengers, called **neurotransmitters** across this space.

There must be enough neurotransmitters for the neuron to relay messages to different parts of the brain. To do the job successfully, the neurotransmitter must stay in the synapse long enough to join onto another neurotransmitter on the surrounding cells. This joining of the neurotransmitter to the receptor is like a key fitting into a lock. When the neurotransmitter (the key) fits into the receptor (the lock) it opens the door for messages to get through.

When the brain is working properly, there are enough neurotransmitters to turn on the cells and deliver the messages effectively. If ADHD is present this process may be inhibited. Messages to put on the brakes, slow down, pay attention or plan, are not be getting through. This results in impulsivity or distractibility.

Brain scans of people with ADHD clearly show that some areas in the brain are underdeveloped. This is mainly in the front of the brain where the organ called the **pre-frontal**

cortex is located, where all executive functions are formed. During the scan the patients were asked to focus and concentrate, it was clear to be seen that parts of their brains did not light up in the expected areas. This explains why people affected by ADHD have trouble with organising, focusing, planning, self-control and learning. There are simply not enough neurotransmitters to activate the neurons in the relevant brain areas.

To correct for this, medications that are used to treat ADHD work by increasing the levels and availability of these neurotransmitters. Scientists have found that there is a system of proteins in each cell that takes the neurotransmitter from the synapse and carries it back inside the specific neuron (cell) that sent it out. These proteins are called transporters. They make up a transporter system at the edge of the cell. People with ADHD have too many of these transporters. This causes the neurotransmitter to be returned to the cell before it has successfully relayed the message to nearby cells.

The problems with neurotransmitters affect some of the brain's functions. They do not affect intelligence, personality or creativity. If you have ADHD you are just as clever and talented as other people.

CONDITIONS THAT OFTEN OCCUR TOGETHER WITH ADHD

(www.aadd.org)
Comorbid conditions are the norm rather than the exception with ADHD. Over 80% of those diagnosed with ADHD will have a co-morbid condition. When I work with clients, I look out for the potential of the client having co-morbid conditions.

- Up to 50% of those with ADHD will have Oppositional Defiance Disorder
- 60% + are affected by Sleep Disorders. It is very common for the circadian rhythm to be out of sync in those with ADHD, which will affect falling asleep, staying asleep, waking up, or a combination of all three.
- Learning disorders like Dyslexia, (up to 76%) Maths, (up to 30%) Written Expression, (65%) Reading Comprehension (52%).
- Anxiety is very common in those with ADHD. Anxiety (42%) and depression (up to 63%) often occur together.
- Obsessive Compulsive Disorder (up to 33%) is another common anxiety disorder common in those with ADHD.
- Co-occurring alcohol abuse disorders ranging up to 45% and drug abuse or dependence ranging up to 30%.
- Mood disorders are common in those with ADHD (38%). This is manifest as persistent irritability and intense or disproportionate anger.
- Up to 40% of those with ADHD will have Hoarding Disorder.
- Up to 50% of those with ADHD exhibit autistic tendencies. 80% those with ASD have ADHD.
- Mood disorders, impulse disorders and any psychiatric disorder are up to 10 times higher in those with ADHD

than in the general population.

From the above statistics it is easy to see how ADHD is linked genetically to other conditions. I have seen that the above conditions can also be more common in the ADHD individual's family, sometimes occurring as traits that are can be clearly observed in family members.

Many people with ADHD who are only diagnosed late in life tend to have high IQs. They learn to cover over and manage their ADHD, until they reach crisis point.

ADHD STATISTICS IN THE UK

ADHD is a worldwide disorder, (Faraone, et al. (2003). As of 2018, about 1.5 million adults in the UK are thought to have ADHD, but only 120,000 are formally diagnosed (ADHD Action). Surveys of children between the ages of 5 and 15 years found that 3.62% of boys and 0.85% of girls had ADHD. In simple terms, this is 3 boys to 1 girl.

The above numbers will change as more research is being done.

ADHD in the UK is shockingly under diagnosed, and under treated. This has crippling and tragic consequences for the person experiencing ADHD as well as their family.

ADHD: BOYS VERSUS GIRLS

Around 5% of children around the world have been diagnosed with ADHD (Polanczyk, et al. 2007). A study found that 60% of these children will continue to live with the condition into adulthood (Harpin, 2005). These children will need lifelong support to manage their ADHD. In the remaining 40% of those diagnosed, as the brain matures the condition will manifest as traits that the person will incorporate into their personality.

More boys than girls are diagnosed with ADHD. Symptoms of ADHD in boys are usually physical, such as excess energy or impulsivity. Boys engage in aggressive and dangerous behaviours more than girls. Boys will externalize their frustrations, so they are far more easily noticed by others in their environment.

More girls than boys have ADD. Girls with ADD tend to display fewer external symptoms. Their difficulties are often missed or mistaken for other conditions such as anxiety and/or depression (Quinn & Madhoo, 2014). Caregivers mistakenly assume that their problems will lessen over time. Girls with undiagnosed ADD will usually suffer from low self-esteem and mental health issues such as anxiety, depression and eating disorders. They are likely to suffer in school, in other social environments and in personal relationships well into their adult lives. Girls with ADD will often fall 'under the radar' as they are not physically disruptive. Many do not get diagnosed at all. These problems if untreated worsen over time.

Girls and women with ADHD are often tragically wrongly diagnosed with depression and anxiety instead of ADD/ADHD. These conditions may be present; however, it is important to understand the ADD/ADHD is usually the dominant condition. In most cases the ADHD condition must be treated first.

Mental health practitioners must fully investigate the subtle symptoms in girls. I have seen with my clients the tragic consequences of women not getting diagnosed early enough, if ever.

ADHD ACROSS THE LIFESPAN

ADHD is a serious condition. Let's look at the ways in which ADHD affects people over the course of their lives.

CHILDREN

Premature birth can activate ADHD genes. Potentially because a baby is experiencing excessive light and sound in what should be a neonatal stage. The ADHD has to be there in first place. Children with ADHD are more vulnerable to bullying or are bullies themselves. Children with ADHD can have a hard time making and keeping friends. Their social impairments often persist into adulthood (Wilens, et al. 2010).

Emotional development in children and teens with ADHD is as much as 30% slower than it is for children without the condition. For example, a 10-year-old with ADHD operates at the maturity level of a 7 year old; a 16 year old beginning driving is using the decision-making skills of an 11 or 12 year old.

For these reasons, children with ADHD are three times more likely to be held back in their studies and in their social skills than their peers. They are far more likely to be home-schooled because most schools are not equipped to help them. (Loe & Feldman, 2007).

Half of all children with ADHD have listening comprehension problems, and are up to 3 times more likely to have problems with expressive language than their neuro-typical peers. Children with ADHD are more likely to bully other children. (Chupetlovska-Anastasova, 2014).

According to a 2018 tweet by child and adolescent psychiatrist Dr. Susan Young, conduct disorder in childhood and ADHD often go together. ADHD related misconduct can persist into adulthood, as evidenced by the 30% of youth and 26% of adult offenders in prisons who present with ADHD symptoms. Most of these offenders (80%) are undiagnosed, and women are less likely to be diagnosed than men.

STUDENTS AND TEENS

About 80 percent of children who need medication for ADHD still need it as teenagers. Teenagers with ADHD commit up to 4 times as many traffic offences than their neuro-typical peers. Teen drivers with ADHD cause car crashes 4 times more often than are their peers without ADHD. They are 7 times more likely to have a second accident. Teenage drivers with ADHD are up to 8 times more likely to have their license suspended or taken away for poor driving behaviour.

Teens with ADHD are twice as likely to have dropped out of high school before finishing their studies. If studies are somehow completed, low grades are common. 45% of teens with ADHD have been suspended. 30% of teens with ADHD have failed or have had to repeat a year of school. The majority of special needs students who are bullied are students diagnosed with Autism Spectrum Disorder and students with ADHD.

They will often find transitioning to college/university much more difficult than their non-ADHD peers. (www.additude.com). In my experience I have seen that they may need one to two gap years in which to mature first. I see daily the dire ramifications of schools and educational settings failing in providing for their ADHD students.

Teens with ADHD are far less likely to attend college/university altogether (Green, et al. 2012). If they do, they may find college studies more difficult than their peers. They are not equipped to advocate for themselves. Due to stress levels, teens with unmanaged ADHD are at greater risk of depression, anxiety and use of alcohol and drugs (Kent, et al. 2011).

I regularly see young teens with ADHD who don't have the necessary life skills for coping in a college environment.

They often fail due to their poor time management skills, problems with concentration, motivation, anxiety, test-taking skills and planning for their studies. It is no surprise that depression and anxiety are common problems in the upper teenage years in those with ADHD.

ADULTS IN THE WORKPLACE

In the workplace, adults with ADHD are two thirds more likely to have been fired from jobs. They are three times more likely to have impulsively quit jobs. They are a third more likely to have chronic employment difficulties. Adults with ADHD are significantly more likely to have changed jobs in a given time frame than their contemporaries. Accordingly, they will often under-earn by a large margin compared to non-ADHD peers.

I have seen how the majority of my ADHD clients do not perform as well as they could in the workplace. Many of my clients have reported being bullied as a result of their challenges that often stem from their ADHD.

It is commonly thought that ADHD is not a fatal condition. Consider the following statistics and draw your own conclusions. Those with ADHD are more likely to engage in dangerous thrill-seeking behaviours. Adults with ADHD are up to 5 times more likely to speed. It is not surprising then at adults with ADHD are nearly 50 percent more likely to be in a serious car crash. Are you surprised then that having ADHD makes you 3 times more likely to be dead by the age of 45? (www.additude.com).

In addition, those with ADHD are far more likely to mismanage their finances and to be dependent on government benefit programs (Altszuler, et al. 2016). I see this a lot with my clients. Those with ADHD often earn far less than they should in relation to their talents and expertise. This massively affects their lives.

RELATIONSHIPS

Those with ADHD are twice as likely to divorce compared to the general population. It is very common for an adult with ADHD to marry another person ADHD, many of my clients have spouses who exhibit similar behaviours and challenges. This obviously leads to families being seriously affected by the hereditary nature of ADHD, leading to lack of family stability, financial difficulties and a volatile emotional environment. All these factors affect the family as a whole, as well as each individual (Wilens, et al. 2010).

Adults with ADHD are 84% more likely to have at least one child with ADHD. They are 50% more likely to have at least two children with ADHD. It is common for parents with ADHD to have relationship problems with their children. Those with ADHD report less stability in relationships and they are less likely to experience the enduring benefits of having a 'best friend' (Chupetlovska, et al. 2014). Many of my clients report being lonely, and having few if any friends.

THE IMPACT OF ADHD IN THE ELDERLY

There are very few statistics in this sector. From personal experience with elderly clients, the ADHD symptoms worsen with age, and are harder to treat effectively. I have seen among my clients that disorganisation and hoarding problems worsen in the aging ADHD population. ADHD in the elderly affects every area of life. I have seen elderly clients with ADHD not investing their finances properly for the future. Depression and anxiety are also more common in the elderly population with ADHD.

Getting diagnosed and receiving appropriate treatment at a younger age greatly impacts how these symptoms manifest in old age.

PART 6
WHAT ARE THE CRITERIA FOR AN ADHD DIAGNOSIS?

WHAT ARE THE CRITERIA FOR AN ADHD DIAGNOSIS?

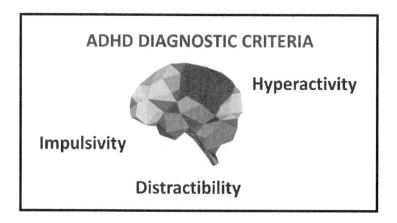

ADHD DIAGNOSTIC CRITERIA

Hyperactivity

Impulsivity

Distractibility

In this chapter you will understand the three core criteria for ADHD, which are written at length in the DSM-5, published by the American Psychiatric Association, and the ICD 10, used by mental health professionals in Europe.

Through learning about ADHD you will come to understand that many characteristics of the condition can actually become strengths when channelled correctly.

The 3 criteria necessary for an ADHD/ADD diagnosis.

1. Hyperactivity
2. Impulsivity
3. Distractibility

HYPERACTIVITY

Hyperactivity manifests itself in two areas:

PHYSICAL RESTLESSNESS

A display of excess energy, especially when bored. This energy is often present as an emotional problem such as low mood or impulsive anger. Fidgeting is one method you might employ to help you focus on boring tasks. Your brain and body are connected. Movements associated with fidgeting actually help your brain maintain focus for learning.

Your brain is wired for excitement. You love new and novel experiences. Life, however is replete with mundane activities. If you have ADHD you will find many tasks daunting or even painful to accomplish. You just haven't got the patience and focus to carry them out. Sleeping, brushing teeth, showering, eating and using the bathroom would typically be too boring to carry out consistently, and on time. Your ADHD brain convinces you to procrastinate until the very last minute, when the deadline looms just ahead. Only then the adrenalin kicks in and pushes you into action mode.

Here is the secret to handling the boring tasks in life:

Learn the necessary skills to establish systems (routines) that will free up your time and mental space. You will find it easier to focus on the important things in your life, and you'll find more time for them.

Restlessness can be an asset. It can be channelled into your passions and dreams, or toward helping others. You probably possess more physical energy and stamina than most people, and it is important to release some of this excess through exercise.

To keep your brain engaged you need to keep on moving. Your abundant energy can work for you instead of against you.

- If your job requires you to sit in one place for long periods of time, consider using a standing desk.
- A quick work out with weights during the day is effective.
- Walking to work would help to get your brain into work focus mode.
- Use your breaks to go for a short jog.

As mentioned before, there is a form of ADHD without hyperactivity. It is called ADD. A person with ADD may appear laid-back or 'chilled'. They don't possess the physical restlessness. They do possess the mental restlessness that will be discussed in the next paragraph.

MENTAL RESTLESSNESS

Your mental restlessness is one of the sources of your endless creative ideas flowing through your brain, bombarding you day and night. This is one source of your inner drive to explore and discover. Do you perceive things that others don't? Do you observe and make connections on a deeper level than others?

You most likely possess more resilience than your peers when faced with setbacks. You are better equipped to persevere and find solutions despite previous failures. You are highly intuitive and grasp concepts quickly, and for this reason you may possess great interpersonal skills.

Some professionals who have embraced their ADHD are rock climbers, explorers, reporters, chefs, hair stylists, comedians and PR managers. Those with ADHD can embrace any professional field, if they know how to handle their ADHD strengths and challenges.

Phil was the creative director of a small film making company. When he saw one of my YouTube videos, he felt that I was speaking directly to him. He asked me for help to calm down his racing thoughts. Phil found it impossible to focus on one project until completion because he kept coming up with more creative ideas.

Phil's brain was on constant overdrive. He complained of extreme fatigue, no doubt due to the overwhelming thoughts bombarding him day and night. Phil got distracted by the goings on around him. His thinking was muddled, and it was difficult to follow him during a conversation as he would jump from topic to topic. He craved true inner calm and peace.

Phil admitted that this problem was causing him great stress and anxiety and was also a source of great tension at home. His wife was fed up with the many unfinished DIY jobs all around the house.

I introduced Phil to some great tools to slow down his brain, including mindfulness. He downloaded a mindfulness app and started practising mindfulness and deep breathing for 10 minutes a day.

I emphasised the importance of finishing tasks. When Phil had a great idea, he got himself into the habit of writing down his idea in a creative diary. He then put the diary aside, to be looked at when he completed his current project.

Phil also started cycling to work. The exercise calmed his racing thoughts, and helped him become more productive.

At home he understood that his DIY projects did not need to be finished to perfection, he understood that they simply needed to be finished to a good enough level. This was particularly difficult for him to implement. We worked through a number of his DIY projects and we discussed various ways to complete those tasks to a good enough level. The books in Phil's study had been piled up all over the place for about three years simply because he didn't have the right screws to adjust the shelves. His wife was beyond fed up with the mess. We brainstormed together, and he came up with three different ideas for screws that he could use to complete the job. At the next session, Phil reported that he had installed the shelves, the books were all neatly stacked in their new homes. His wife was delighted.

When a project was finally completed, he used to agonise over how he could have done it better. I introduced him to the 'done perfect' idea. Once a project was completed, then it was 'perfect', and it was time to focus onwards...

After a few weeks of focusing on task completion, Phil told me that he felt more inner peace and grounding.

Nathan was plagued with self-doubt. He was bright but complained that he was constantly tormented by his creative brain, which constantly bombarded him with new ideas. This paralysed him with indecision and overwhelm. He was 35 and had not yet brought to fruition any of his creative plans.

He watched with envy as those he knew, who were far less capable than him, reached their goals in life. This bothered him greatly. After his first session, his first homework assignment was to write down as many of his creative ideas as he could think of. Every time a creative idea entered his consciousness, he had to write it down. At the next session I asked him to focus on one idea and take the necessary steps to actualise it. Nathan found this excruciatingly difficult.

I explained to him the following parable:

Imagine you are camping out in the countryside, and you come across a stream with beautiful multi-coloured fish swimming along. You want to catch some fish for your lunch. You only need to catch one fish. When it is time for dinner, you will go back and catch another fish.

I explained to Nathan that his ideas would keep on swimming down the stream of his consciousness. He only needed to catch one idea, and take the steps to bring it to completion. Nathan managed to complete one goal, and then move on to the next. He reported feeling more productive and energetic than he had ever felt in his life.

IMPULSIVITY

When people hear the term ADHD, they think of the inability to focus for extended lengths of time. The core challenge however, is regulating emotions and impulses. Your ADHD brain is more susceptible to impulsivity. Behaviours such as blurting out comments, or impulsive spending are typical. Redirect your impulsive urges. If saying 'no' to yourself is too hard, simply say 'yes' to something else and wait for the first craving to pass. Racing drivers, test pilots, entrepreneurs, media producers, talk show hosts, and artists have all harnessed their 'impulsivity' towards successful careers.

Remember that you will find boring tasks very difficult to do. Harness your impulsivity to make the task creative and exciting. Your impulsivity is a gift that you have a responsibility to harness in a positive way.

On a personal note, I managed to get this book completed by harnessing my trait of impulsivity. I had the idea to write this book, and jumped in right away. Once I had gotten over the exciting part of writing the book, I needed to wade through the horribly boring task of proofreading and checking, (6 times!) I got this done by jumping from one part of the book to the other, starting from the centre of the book and working outwards. I worked in half hour increments, and changed the environment that I worked in. These simple methods kept my brain buzzing and helped me deal with the overwhelmingly boring yet vital task of editing, proof reading and finishing this book.

Being impulsive is an important trait for action. If you possess this trait, you have the ability to be brave and step up to the task, when you believe it is the right thing to do. Impulsivity is the root of the classic pioneer.

Alice was a single mother with an adult son who had ADHD. Pete was still living at home, with no job and nothing to do. He was a very frustrated young man. She was overwhelmed and deeply worried about what the future would bring. Nicola wanted help to improve her relationship with Pete.

When Alice first started coaching, she learned about the symptoms of ADHD. She understood how her lack of empathy for his condition had contributed to the breakdown in their relationship. She would repeatedly get upset that he didn't listen to her, giving no eye contact, and he would fidget with small items when she spoke to him.

I explained to her that many people who have ADHD may need to fidget with a small item to help them focus on every day conversations. When a person with ADHD processes new information, they may find it difficult to make eye contact. Alice felt terrible when she recalled how she used to insist that Pete stop fidgeting, and look her in the face. I explained to her the importance of self-forgiveness. She had done the best with the tools she had had at the time.

Alice learned tools to help her diffuse the tension between her and Pete. She learned how to recognise her body's signs when she was getting angry, which helped her be silent and refrain from answering back when Pete got upset. She learned how to calm herself down when tensions did arise.

Alice felt she had finally found the tools she had been lacking. I supported her in implementing those tools between sessions. As a result, she felt much happier with herself.

These tools helped Alice make improvements in many other areas of her life. Here is her testimonial after a particularly gruelling week.

"My elderly father was admitted into hospital for a minor operation. I spent two weeks running back and forth from the hospital to my Mum's home, then to my own home. I was supporting my Dad in hospital, who hardly spoke any English, and supporting my elderly mum in running her home. I also had to keep my own home running smoothly.

"In the past I would have verbally let out my stress on family members without thinking. I can honestly say that in those two weeks I did not have one meltdown. I feel calm and in control. I understand that my hypofocusing powers, being able to keep so many balls juggling in the air, have been my biggest strength in this situation. I have put myself first, by still attending the gym every morning, even if it was for a shorter workout, and practising my ten minute daily mindfulness routine. Putting my self-care first has helped me focus on my

Clients regularly make great changes in life areas that they haven't even worked on in the coaching sessions. This is because when one improves on one executive function it has a direct effect on the other executive functions.

This is Nicola's story. She was in coaching for five months practising self-awareness and emotional self-regulation.

Nicola had a sister-in-law, Alex, with whom she didn't get on very well. Alex was a high-flying executive who earned over two million a year. Nicola was employed as a desk clerk at her local post office. She felt intimidated by Alex. During a recent conversation, Alex made a remark that deeply hurt Nicola. She felt that Alex seriously crossed her boundaries. She related that a couple of days after the incident she invited Alex out for a drink. Nicola was scared out of her wits but she calmly yet assertively stated her thoughts about Alex's remarks. Alex understood that her comments had been out of place. She apologised.

Nicola related that in all her 54 years she had never managed to assert herself in a calm and forthright manner. Had she followed her regular behaviour pattern she would have simply shut down or more likely, exploded in anger at a later time. This moment of brave assertiveness was a major achievement for her. She felt five feet taller. She gained confidence that she could face future challenges successfully.

DISTRACTIBILITY

So many people who are assessed for ADHD are still not getting a correct ADHD diagnosis. This is because it is commonly thought that if you can focus or concentrate then you do not have ADHD. This is not true.

If you have ADHD you can focus very well on the topics that interest you. As mentioned earlier in the book, you have super strong focus powers. You can even focus for far longer than other people. This is only true if what you are focusing on is interesting for you.

The problem with focus and attention is that you pay attention to far too many things at once. You find it difficult to focus your attention to only one thing at a time. Your many thoughts bombard you and torment you and don't give you rest. You find it difficult to prioritise your tasks and get things done.

With the right skills you can learn to slow down your thoughts, prioritise, and focus on one task at a time.

The most enlightening idea during Peter's six months of coaching was learned to develop his ability to stay on task till completion. Initially, he found this impossible to do. He found that physical movement fired up his brain, and helped him focus. He learned to use his distractibility strength to sprint from task to task in rapid fire succession. He gave himself permission to shift focus within a few tasks, but to make sure to finish them, and this helped keep up his interest.

GET A DIAGNOSIS

The first step toward your ADHD treatment is to get a diagnosis. A diagnosis doesn't define you. It simply puts your symptoms into a labelled box. After the diagnosis you are still the same creative, resourceful person as before. Your diagnosis will open doors for appropriate help and support.

Untreated ADHD impacts all areas of life, and can be fatal. Those with ADHD say that they see their own potential and have a deep desire to fulfil their many goals but get so frustrated as they sense an internal block. This block is real. It is the developmental delay associated with ADHD.

So much can be done to help those with ADHD. Getting a diagnosis as early as possible helps to prevent so much emotional damage that sets in with years of failure.

The ADHD situation is slowly changing in the UK. I personally know many practitioners and doctors who are working tirelessly to improve the situation in the UK. These courageous individuals and groups are challenging the government to overhaul and quicken the diagnostic process and treatment for patients.

So many clients tell me that they don't need to get a diagnosis. They just need to work on the symptoms. While I understand them, I always advocate getting a diagnosis.

Consider the following:

Firstly, you may have a totally different condition that needs addressing. Secondly, if you live in the UK, and you have an ADHD diagnosis you will have access to government funding to help you manage your ADHD at home and at work. Thirdly, please understand that getting a diagnosis, labels your symptoms, not yourself. ADHD does not affect your intelligence levels. Professionals agree that getting a diagnosis helps you to accept your situation and move on. Until you do so, you will be held back.

In my experience the clients that got assessed and received a diagnosis moved further towards their goals than those who didn't go down the route to get assessed.

THE FIVE STAGES OF ACCEPTANCE

When you receive an ADHD diagnosis for yourself or a loved one there may be an initial period of relief or euphoria. Your symptoms have a name, you are not crazy or lazy! But once these feelings start to wear off you may start to experience other emotions.
Below are five stages of emotion that you will most likely go through:

1. Denial and isolation
2. Anger
3. Resentment
4. Depression
5. Acceptance

You don't necessarily go through the stages in the above order, or even experience all of the stages. It is common to move forward and backwards from one to the other, even in the course of one day. Any emotion that you may be feeling in relation to your ADHD diagnosis, whether positive or negative, is acceptable. You may wish to process your feelings with a therapist in order to make sense of your inner experiences.

HOW DO YOU GET YOURSELF ASSESSED FOR ADHD?

You will have likely read an article or seen something in the news about ADHD. You think that you may have ADHD. You want to get a diagnosis.

Here are some pointers to help you along your journey. To get an ADHD diagnosis in the UK you will need to be assessed by a qualified adult ADHD specialist such as an ADHD psychiatrist. Sadly the process may not be that smooth for you. This is due in large part to the total ignorance of GPs and even specialist ADHD professionals about the true nature of ADHD in adults. You may need to push through some barriers until you get yourself referred and then seen by an ADHD specialist.

GETTING AN NHS ADHD DIAGNOSIS

In England and Wales, adult diagnosis and treatment is based on the NICE Guidelines which were published in September 2008, prior to that date, the NHS did not recognise adult ADHD. There is no consistent ADHD procedure across the UK. Some regions have better services and shorter waiting lists than others. Tragically in some areas there is no ADHD adult service.

I tell my clients that they need to prepare well before their 10-minute GP appointment. They should take along the ICD 10 diagnostic criteria, with the relevant symptoms circled, and to have some 'extreme' instances of how they think their ADHD has impacted them.

I tell my clients that if the GP refuses to refer them to an ADHD specialist they should make another appointment with another GP in the practise and repeat the process. If the GP still refuses to refer, I advise my clients to change GPs or practice. It is handy to take along a copy of the NICE Guidelines so that if necessary you can show that the NHS fully supports adult diagnosis and ADHD.

If your GP agrees to refer you further, then please do follow up with the GP a week after the appointment

If you have gotten past this hurdle the next step is that your GP will refer the you to a community mental health team, who in turn can make the referral to the ADHD specialist psychiatrist. Or your GP could refer you directly to the ADHD specialist team.

The NHS assessment will be free, but you may have to wait an awfully long time.

GETTING A PRIVATE ADHD DIAGNOSIS

The private route is the quickest and least painful. There are many independent psychiatrists who offer a good ADHD assessment and you can be seen within a week. A word of warning here, just because you are paying for your assessment will not guarantee a good treatment plan. Sadly, so many clients have told me shocking stories of their awful experiences with private ADHD specialists. Choose carefully. Only go to a recommended ADHD specialist.

Please be aware that the symptoms of women with ADHD differ greatly from those of men with ADHD. Anxiety and depression are the most common ADHD symptoms. So many clients tell me their story how they were misdiagnosed with anxiety or depression or worse, and the underlying root condition, their ADHD was not even looked for.

Find a good psychiatrist who will screen you for comorbidities. Over 80% of those with ADHD have a second comorbid condition.

I prefer the shared care route. The ADHD medications are expensive and you will have to pay for them the first time your psychiatrist prescribes them to you. After this you can ask your GP to prescribe the medications on the NHS. As your psychiatrist to write to your GP and create a shared care agreement. This means that your psychiatrist takes the responsibility and determines what the GP will prescribe for you. Once this has been set up, your only ongoing costs will be a 6 monthly or annual visit/call with your private psychiatrist.

PART 7
UNLOCK YOUR ADHD SUPER POWERS

UNLOCK YOUR ADHD SUPERPOWERS

In many cultures ADHD is not seen as a disorder. It is viewed as a personality type. If you truly want success you simply need to channel your ADHD traits to serve you, and your life goals.

Your ADHD deficits are a smokescreen covering up your strengths. Most of my clients approach me because they want help to manage their deficits. They have lost hope in discovering their strengths. Many don't even believe that they have strengths. This chapter will explore some of the strengths that you possess in abundance. Yes, you do! If you truly want success you simply need to channel your ADHD (read deficits) to serve you and your life goals. Recognising your strengths and understanding how to harness them in the appropriate way will open the gateway to your success.

ADHD is not an illness. It is not something to shy away from, it is not something to hide. ADHD is a trait, not a disability. When managed correctly, it can become a huge asset; a superpower that will help you achieve the unimaginable.

Your ADHD brain is like a powerful racing car with bicycle brakes. You need tools to learn how to strengthen your brakes in order to function at your optimum best.

There have been many famous people over the course of history who might have had ADHD.

- Albert Einstein was one of the greatest contributors to modern day science.
- Frank Lloyd Wright was one of the most preeminent architects of the 20th century.
- Vincent Van Gogh painted some of the most highly valued paintings hanging in art museums worldwide.
- Mozart created over 600 masterpieces in his short life.
- Abraham Lincoln led the USA at a time of political

unrest, and delivered the Gettysburg address, which is still quoted today.

Another way of describing hypofocusing is mind-wandering. Many people with ADHD relate that they feel a strong internal pull to drift away from intense focus. One client called it her mind at play. It is your brain's default mode; the place where it goes to chill when working at some mental task. If you have ADHD it is absolutely vital to give your brain time for this because it will enable you to focus better in the long run. You will need to find suitable methods to get yourself back into regular focus mode when necessary. Do you find transitions difficult? Mind-wandering is the built-in mechanism for managing daily transitions.

Vera worked part-time in a social media marketing company. Her creative talents were a great asset to her company. Her boss wanted to give her a promotion but Vera was afraid. For her, the daily transition from work to home was daunting. She had many commitments at home and struggled to focus on them. How would she manage with the increased work load?

When explaining the idea of mind-wandering I stressed that her brain needed some time to transition from work mode to home mode. I encouraged her when she got home after work to just sit and do nothing for a while. Vera needed some convincing as she felt that sitting on the couch and doing nothing was a total waste of time.

She tried it for a week and was astonished at the results. Vera reported that she was getting more done at home, feeling more positive at work, and was suffering less from the severe headaches that had plagued her since age twelve.

It is so important to give yourself breaks during the course of the day to simply do nothing. So many clients tell me that in the evening they just crash out on the couch for ages, (1-2 hours). Does this ever happen to you in a similar form? This is your brain telling you that it has focused too hard during the day. It is your brain protesting at being forced to focus so intensely without a break!

When you leave a field to lie fallow the nutrients in the earth replenish themselves for a better crop yield in the future. When you simply sit and do nothing for 5-10 minutes a couple of times a day, you are allowing your brain to replenish its focus powers to serve you better for the rest of the day. This is one of the components to living a balanced life.

Eva, a coaching client was a young mum. She found it so terribly difficult and painfully boring to sit and play with her young children for longer than 5 minutes. When I explained to her the idea of mind-wandering, she learned to look forward to her playing time with her children. Every Sunday morning, she sat with her kids for a longer length of time, and played with them on the floor. She learned to look forward to this time in her week. She knew that every week without fail, as she would play with them, and her mind simply wandered, an insight or a solution to a current problem would usually fall into her consciousness.

UNLOCK YOUR TALENTS

Do you look at the world in an innovative way? Do you find solutions to problems that were previously deemed unsolvable?

You are motivated by your own inner deadlines and not by external factors. Your inner values mean a lot to you. They can motivate you far more effectively than deadlines enforced on you by others.

You believe in your ideas independently, even when others criticise them. You often prove yourself right by producing brilliant work. Many companies are looking for people like you. Neurodiversity is becoming increasingly popular for companies wanting to grow and expand.

It is likely that many people do not understand you or even get to know you properly. This can be incredibly lonely and painful. It is vital that you make a concerted effort to spend time with people who do understand you, and who share similar creative energy as you.

Push through your challenges. You are doubtless made of strong stuff. Your resilience will help you to learn from mistakes and forge ahead to reach your goals. Try delegating the more 'boring' aspects of your projects to others, so that you can focus on the tasks you excel in.

I met a middle-aged woman who had ADHD. She was an international lecturer. I asked her how she managed her paperwork. "What paperwork?" was her reply. She received her bills and bank statements online. Any important paperwork was delegated to her son to take care of. She proudly proclaimed her home 'Paperwork free!' This is a woman whose awareness of her limitations helps her to get ahead in life.

DISCOVER YOUR INNATE STRENGTHS

Your creativity is your impulsivity turned the right way around...

The chart below displays the most common executive functions and ADHD deficits. The column on the right shows the positive, 'strength' perspective. You have the power to convert your past pain and struggles into present and future strengths.

CHALLENGE	STRENGTH
1 – Focus challenges You have difficulty focusing on mundane or boring tasks.	You can keep your focus on many things at once. You can sustain focus for long time periods on what interests you. You see potential and possibilities. Distractions help you access your intuition.
2 – Poor processing This affects your thought, clarity and decision-making skills.	You connect random ideas to form a plan unique to you. You can start anew any time – you are not constrained by past judgements. You develop new, innovative ways to create and link memory associations. You see the big picture where others see the fine details.

3 – Low self-awareness and self-esteem You may be super aware of other people's strengths, yet show poor awareness of your own talents, interests, passions and desires. You may be unaware how much your actions affect those in your environment	You are easy going. You have the ability to be highly tolerant of difficult situations. You have a strong desire to learn about yourself and contribute to the world. You are open to change.
4- Physical restlessness (Physical hyperactivity) You have excess restless energy, especially when bored or not engaged.	You thrive on change and embrace excitement. You notice things that others don't. You are incredibly energetic and full of life. You are driven and open to risk-taking. You are an extremely hard worker when the work is in line with your values. You are willing to continue trying despite past failures.
5 – Mental restlessness (Cognitive hyperactivity) You experience nonstop ideas/connections, as well as nonstop thoughts in rapid-fire succession.	You are constantly looking for new ideas for stimulation. People say you are an 'idea machine'. You intuitively leap into new projects when you sense this is the right thing to do, leaving others far behind.

6 – Poor time management You may have a weak concept of time, with no frame of reference for determining how long it will take to do a task.	You live through intuitive time flow and are not constrained by time. You have your own unique internal organisation method that only you understand.
7 – Overwhelm shutdown You experience nonstop thoughts or stimuli that manifest in anxiety or excessive worry, which leads to an inability to take action.	You intuitively know when to self-protect and take the necessary steps to do this.
8 – Poor self-regulation (spending, blurting, overeating) You may be unable to regulate or manage reactions and emotions. You experience boredom and impatience more often than others.	You are quick and spontaneous. Your responses are genuine. You are willing to take risks. You are a visionary.
9 – Procrastination You push off decisions and starting projects.	You have high standards and expectations of yourself. You take time over your work and analyse the situation from all angles.
10 – Anger You find it challenging to control or manage your outbursts of anger. You may exhibit flash anger.	You react quickly in a given situation. You have intense energy and enthusiasm. When you understand what your trigger points are you can educate yourself about possible areas of growth.

11 – Deep, dark thoughts Your brain can become fixated on negative thoughts that immobilise and paralyse you.	You can develop detailed complex systems and processes. You can utilize your intense concentration powers in your area of interest. You possess a vivid imagination.
12 – Incompletions You may exhibit weak follow-through, especially in your areas of disinterest or overwhelm.	You work well to deadlines if the project resonates with your values. You thrive on carrying through a project in a short amount of time, like a sprinter running a race. In your areas of passion, you are extremely productive.
13 – Poor productivity under pressure You feel you have poor stress management skills.	You thrive in safe partnerships. Internal deadlines drive you.
14 – Black and white thinking Your all-or-nothing thinking inhibits you from taking action. Your perfectionism often paralyses your progress.	You are detailed and meticulous about what you value.
15 -Physical and emotional sensitivities Hypersensitivity to your environment may interfere with your life efficiency.	You are sensitive, emotive and empathic. You may be charismatic due to your deep awareness of the emotional state of those around you.

16 – **Executive function/dysfunction** You have a poor working memory, struggle with prioritisation, planning and self-regulation.	You are uninhibited and live in the moment. You are willing to try something in front of a group. When you want to complete a project, you will stick with it until it is done. You compensate for your executive function deficits by using your emotions to guide you.

CONNECT WITH YOUR CREATIVITY EVERY SINGLE DAY

To live successfully with your ADHD, you must find an outlet for your energy every day, no matter what! Spend focused time doing the activities you love. Make time for yourself, and you will feel refreshed and vibrant. Most importantly, when life hits, as it does, you will be more likely to bounce back quicker, and handle life with more resilience.

Rosie and I spent only two coaching sessions together, which led to various insights. Rosie, a dental receptionist, was on medication to manage her depression. She started coaching because she wanted help to improve her performance at work. She was overwhelmed with torment at her poor performance. Not surprisingly she had a poor self-image. She believed she was incompetent and was grappling with deep feelings of shame.

Rosie hated her job. She hated sorting and filing patient records. Sorting and filing were a large part of her job and she didn't understand how she kept on messing up. Rosie often forgot to give over important messages to colleagues, with terribly embarrassing results. She was overwhelmed, ashamed and grappled with feelings of uselessness. Her director was fed up with her incompetence.

Rosie desperately wanted help managing her current job successfully.

Through coaching she discovered her strengths and her talents. This was a really difficult thing to do, as she had never paid attention to this before. She understood that her current job was a total misfit for her nature.

Rosie discovered that she loved to organise events. She loved being in nature. She loved animals. She realised that her current job was the wrong fit for her. Through coaching she became empowered to take that big step and leave.

Rosie volunteered at a local animal sanctuary and started spending time in nature. I didn't hear from her for a while, and hoped things were going well.

Rosie called me a couple of months later. She said that this was the first time she felt so energised and positive in her life. Because of the self-knowledge she had gained through our coaching sessions, her depression had lifted, and her doctor had reduced her dose of anti-depressants. She told me that she had enrolled to train as a wilderness instructor.

Your ADHD is your biggest strength, and in the right environment and support you can succeed beyond your wildest dreams.

PART 8
YOUR SUCCESSFUL LIFE
WITH YOUR ADHD

ADHD PILLS

In this section you will read about common ADHD treatments. The purpose of this section is to make you aware of the many forms of treatment for your ADHD. It is vital that you do further research to find out more about the treatments you may be interested in.

This section provides a general overview of ADHD medication, the first line of conventional treatment for ADHD. This section is intended to jump start your research and point you in the right direction.

Getting an ADHD diagnosis opens the doors for treatment. Your ADHD does not define who you are; your ADHD is simply another feature of your unique personality.

In the UK, there is unfortunately still a great stigma regarding ADHD and administering ADHD medications. There has been a lot of negative publicity associated with ADHD medications. Many people still believe that they are risky and have negative side-effects. This attitude is largely based on ignorance. Spreading these lies does a huge disservice to the public and stops many people from getting the treatment they need. Many studies have concluded that ADHD medications are safe to use. The ADHD medications are the first line of treatment for ADHD. ADHD medications, when they are working in your brain, compensate for the biological problem at the root of your ADHD. The medications work well for an overwhelming majority of the population, with most reporting substantial improvements in quality of life.

It may take you some time to find the right medication and the correct dose. Keep on trying until you do. Each case, of course, must be judged on its own merits, as each individual reacts differently to medication. You may need to try out several different types and brands until you find one that works for you.

There is a misconception that ADHD stimulant medications are addictive. When administered responsibly, ADHD medications are not addictive. They actually help those with ADHD manage their addictions. 16 studies have been conducted in this area and found no connection between taking ADHD medication and substance abuse later on in life. One study found a greater risk, but the results were not analysed correctly. (Barkley 2010). The risk of addiction to street drugs in many people with untreated ADHD is very high.

It is well known that there is a higher incidence of smoking among those with unmedicated ADHD. Nicotine is a known stimulant, and may act on the brain in similar ways to ADHD medication. Nicotine may help some smokers with ADHD compensate for their low levels of attention, focus, self-control, and working memory. This may be why those with ADHD are at a higher risk of smoking because of the beneficial effects of nicotine on the ADHD brain.

Various studies have found that those with ADHD who previously smoked, and are currently on ADHD medication, very often quit smoking. The brain doesn't need the beneficial effects of nicotine anymore, as it is getting it from the ADHD medication. More research needs to be done in this area.

Please consider the following question carefully:

You have only one life to live. Why should you live a more difficult life just because you have ADHD?

In the USA, where ADHD medication is more widely accepted, there are still far too many people falling through the cracks and not accessing diagnosis and treatment. Many of my clients have children with ADHD. They are often hesitant to give the meds to their child. My experience has shown that the meds are massively powerful in helping students focus and get through school. If your child has ADHD and has been prescribed medication just be thankful that there is a tool that has the potential to help your child get through their studies.

Tom, aged eight, had been diagnosed with ADHD. His dad, Richard, insisted that the ADHD meds were poison and he would never give them to his son. Richard looked into alternative therapies for Tom to help him focus and manage his temper. They worked but with only partial success. When Tom was ten years old, Richard received a call from the school office that Tom had been suspended. In a fit of rage he had hit a teacher and broken some school equipment. Richard sought help from Tom's ADHD coach, who advised him to follow the route of ADHD medication. With much reluctance, Richard agreed to try it; if this would help Tom get through school then so be it.

The meds really helped Tom to focus and stay calm. He still needed help with time management and organisation skills. When the meds were working in his body he was more receptive to the tools that he was learning, and better able to implement them in his life.

ADHD SKILLS

There are many forms of treatment that work well with ADHD. Here is a list of some of the most common ones. The success of each treatment will differ widely from person to person, with varying factors such as environment, and individual commitment.

CBT

Cognitive Behavioral Therapy (CBT) is a form of therapy that has proven successful in treating those with ADHD (Knouse, 2010). When combined with ADHD medication it has been even more effective.

CBT, originally developed by Albert Ellis in the 1950s, was called Rational Emotive Behaviour Therapy. It was then revised and called Cognitive Therapy by Aaron T. Beck in the 1960s. CBT targets thoughts, feelings and beliefs, and how the client can achieve emotional self-regulation.

I would like to put in a word of caution here. If you have ADHD it is vital that you find a CBT practitioner who understands your ADHD related challenges. I have heard too many stories from clients who have reported that CBT has not been as effective as it could be simply because the practitioner lacked the right ADHD awareness and understanding. The tools were therefore not adapted to suit their needs. Only use a practitioner who in known to understand ADHD, and the challenges associated with it.

DBT

DBT, or Dialectical Behaviour Therapy was conceived in the 1980s by Marsha Linehan, Ph.D., Professor of Psychology at the University of Washington and founder of The Linehan Institute. DBT was originally developed to treat those with Borderline Personality Disorder, and was designed to stand up to the intense emotions and physical reactions associated with BPD.

BPD is a mental health illness. It is the inability to manage and modulate one's emotions. Sometimes the person with BPD will have serious problems with all relationships, sometimes only just with one. Many symptoms of BPD overlap with the emotional self-regulation challenges associated with ADHD. More research is being carried out to understand how this works. DBT or Dialectical Behaviour Therapy, is gaining popularity as a viable treatment for ADHD.

I am a great advocate of DBT as it is designed to help clients understand and manage their emotions.

ADHD COACHING

Successful ADHD management is "Pills and Skills." Unmanaged ADHD affects every area of life. ADHD coaching complements ADHD medications. (Prevatt, et al. 2015), (Field, et al. 2010), (Ferrin, et al. 2016). ADHD medication only manages up to 50% of ADHD symptoms. The remaining 50% needs to be addressed through ADHD coaching. This is specific coaching that teaches the ADHD client the life skills that they need in order to succeed with their ADHD.

Every person diagnosed with ADHD needs some aspect of life skills training and support to compensate for their executive function deficits. When the ADHD sufferer lives life catching up from one self-made crisis to another, they may end up with serious emotional issues that need to be therapy. ADHD coaching support must be offered first before therapy. An expert ADHD coach will challenge their client to come out of his/her comfort zone, move forward and put into action the tools at their own pace.

When Mark started coaching, he was hyperfocused on his weaknesses. His negative focus pulled him into a vortex of self-blame and inaction. Through coaching he learned to challenge his beliefs, and totally transform his self-image. While still aware of his deficits, he now walks with his head held high due to his deep awareness of his strengths. He is in the process of setting up his own software company, a dream he has come to actualise through coaching.

PROFESSIONAL ORGANISING

Hiring a professional organiser to teach you how to de-clutter and organise yourself (and your papers...) is a great move forward. A professional organiser will be very beneficial in managing the practical aspects of your ADHD. An organised home leads to an organised mind; an organised mind leads to organised goals and an organised business. Find a professional organiser who understands ADHD.

Amy, a stay-at-home mum with four children, called our team desperately seeking help getting her papers organised. She felt totally overwhelmed by her papers, and admitted having lost over £3,000 in benefits due to a misplaced document.

Through the coaching sessions Amy learnt how to sort and store her papers, and how to maintain her newfound system. Amy was so empowered with the changes that she bravely applied for a part-time job and got the position.

Phil had been diagnosed with ADD and was training to become a pharmacist. He found the meds very helpful and took them every day at the same time. While they were active they helped him to focus and he got much more done. He managed to complete his studies.

Sometime later, due to the nature of his job he had an enormous amount of paperwork, including reports, to write up and sort. While the meds were excellent, they did not teach him how to organise his paperwork. He turned to a professional organiser to successfully learn those skills.

NEUROFEEDBACK

This therapy can be very beneficial in those people who take well to it. Neurofeedback helps with concentration and focus, attention and hyperactivity. Medication may have a bigger initial effect, whereas the changes resulting from neurofeedback may be experienced over a more extended period of time. (Fernandez, et al. 2017), (Steiner, et al. 2013).

OCCUPATIONAL THERAPY

Many people, including children with ADHD, suffer from sensory sensitivities. You may benefit from the assistance of an occupational therapist, who would put together an individually planned 'sensory diet' that would provide you with the focus and stimulation you need to keep you alert and focused as you go through your day. The therapist may provide you with different tools to use at different times of the day, based on your schedule and personal tendencies.

IMPROVED DIET

According to the International Society for Nutritional Psychiatry research, a healthy diet is essential for managing ADHD. I have seen the great benefits of a balanced diet, and eating three set meals a day has on clients' wellbeing and focus.

There are conflicting views that ADHD is caused by diet or nutritional problems. However, certain foods have been shown to worsen ADHD symptoms. Cutting out white flour and sugar may help to sharpen the mind and sustain energy. Eating more healthfully will make you feel lighter and more positive about yourself. This will have a direct impact on your life. Eat three meals a day at regular intervals. Avoid caffeine after 3:00 pm as this may interfere with your sleep.

Some people with ADHD may be sensitive to food colourings and preservatives. The Mayo Clinic lists the following colourings and preservatives that may increase hyperactive behaviour in children and adults.

- Sodium benzoate, often found in carbonated drinks, salad dressings and fruit juice products.
- Sunset yellow found in breadcrumbs, cereal, sweets, icing and soft drinks.
- Quinoline yellow found in juices, sorbets and smoked haddock.
- Tartrazine found in foods such as pickles, cereal, granola bars and yogurt.
- Allura red found in soft drinks, children's medications, gelatin desserts and ice cream.

Like most things in life, moderation is the way to go. Establishing good nutritional habits can truly be life-changing.

Flora started coaching to learn some tools to help her when she felt overwhelmed and anxious.

During the first session she set her goals - she really wanted help with losing weight and keeping it off. Flora needed to lose three stone as her doctor had warned her that her excess weight was affecting her health. She was terrified that she would die young, as her mother had done, due to complications from being overweight. This fear kept her up at night. She was deeply ashamed of her self-image.

Over the years she had seen a number of nutritionists to help her lose weight, with little success. They had told her what changes to make in her life, but had not guided her how to go about it. This time she was determined to succeed. I worked with her to set up a menu plan and master shopping list that worked with her personality and lifestyle. We broke down the steps and worked at her pace Flora learned how to find the time to prepare her meals.

Flora felt intense relief. It was a slow process as Flora had never created menu plans before in her life. Meals had always been ad hoc – consisting of whatever she had in the house, or take-away food, which was not the healthiest option.

It took time for Flora to integrate her new actions into solid habits. Flora felt energised and more focused. She realised that her short-term goal for healthy eating was to have more energy and focus, the weight would come off little by little.

Flora's family benefitted from her new menu system. Maria, her teenage daughter, suffered from mood fluctuations. With the healthier eating changes in place her moods stabilised.

She felt that she now had the tools and support she needed to reach her goals. Flora didn't have to hide herself from the world anymore. She sensed her true potential unfolding.

SUPPLEMENTS

There is some evidence that shows herbal supplements to be somewhat effective. This varies from person to person so it is critical to always consult with your doctor before including any supplements in your diet. Omega 3 fish oils may be helpful in managing some ADHD symptoms. Supplementing with Omega 3s can improve attention and behaviour, as well as sleep patterns.

Too many clients waste so much money on supplements and all sorts of new-fangled ideas that promise to help them in a very short amount of time. I believe there are no magic solutions. Success comes through work and consistent effort. Be very cautious before you take on any new supplement or treatment plan that promises you instant results.

LIMIT ALCOHOL CONSUMPTION

The dangers of alcohol abuse and brain damage in those with ADHD are startling. ADHD often occurs together with alcohol or drug addiction (Smith, et al. 2002). I have seen this many times with clients. The rate of ADHD is at least 25% among patients receiving treatment for alcohol or drug addiction, and 20 to 50% of adults diagnosed with ADHD meet criteria for alcohol or drug addiction. Furthermore, the rate of ADHD may be as high as 50% in high–risk populations. The good news is that proper treatment with ADHD medications reduces the risk of substance abuse by 85%. Read that again. The good news is that proper treatment with ADHD medications reduces the risk of substance abuse by 85 percent.

SLEEP INTERVENTIONS

The circadian rhythm can be out of whack in people with ADHD. When this happens the sleep hormone melatonin doesn't get released at the right time. This can cause sleep problems. It is crucial that those suffering from sleep problems seek help in implementing regular fixed hours of sleep. Lack of sleep leads to hazy thinking, low moods and lack of clarity.
Some common sleep problems in those with ADHD are:

- Difficulty falling and staying asleep
- Restless sleep
- Nightmares/disturbing dreams
- Not enough sleep and serious sleep deficit
- Difficulty winding down at bedtime
- Difficulty waking up in the morning at a regular time
- Needing more sleep than the average person
- Restless leg syndrome (Cortese, et al. 2008)
- Those with ADHD may be wired to be more alert at night

Basic sleep interventions:

- Create a regular sleep routine. Go to bed and get up at the same time every day, even on weekends.
- Take time to relax every evening.
- Get plenty of physical exercise during the day. This helps with sleep.
- Consider getting a daytime light to brighten the room in the mornings to slowly shift the circadian rhythm.
- Omega three supplements may help. Always consult your doctor before taking supplements.

Barry wanted help regulating his sleep patterns. He had tried to help himself for several years, with poor results. He knew that a good sleep routine was at the root of his success, and he was determined to overcome his challenge. Most evenings, before he knew it, it was 2:00 am before he was able to get into bed. He was perplexed where the time went every evening. I encouraged him to keep a sleep diary, documenting the activities he did every evening.

After a while he realised that his problem wasn't falling asleep, it was transitioning from daytime mode to sleep mode. We set up some simple routines that encouraged his brain to transition easily from one time frame to the next.

We identified and managed the distractions that stopped him from getting to bed. Barry set up a sleep routine. It took about six months to implement the changes. Slowly and steadily, Barry started going to sleep earlier. As his natural bedtime shifted, he started waking up earlier in the mornings. He felt energised and more self-confident, which greatly impacted both his work and home life.

MINDFULNESS

Mindfulness has been around for a very long time. In the last ten years its benefits have become more widely recognised (Mitchell, et al. 2015). Mindfulness is a form of self-awareness and focus training. Practising mindfulness improves your ability to focus. Your brain can rewire itself through any behaviour that you reinforce through repetition.

Deep inside you there is a voice; the voice of your soul. If you are receptive, you will hear its message. The problem is that the soul voice is all too often drowned out by the buzz of technology and life's pastimes. If you slow down and listen, it will give you excellent advice as it knows you very, very well!

Mindfulness utilises the power of breathing. The purpose of breathing is to get oxygen to your brain for optimal efficiency. Breathing brings clean oxygen from the air into your body and energises you. When you breathe out you eliminate harmful carbon dioxide. Every cell in your body needs oxygen in order to function properly. Brain cells are particularly sensitive to oxygen levels; they will start to die within four minutes of being deprived of oxygen.

When you have a stressful reaction, your breathing becomes shallow. Shallow breathing is inefficient as the oxygen that normally travels to the brain is significantly reduced. As a result you will become more irritable, impulsive and confused.

Stop what you are doing and breathe in slowly and deeply through your diaphragm. Feel your stomach rising and falling a couple of times. There, you have started on your mindful journey; it really is that simple.

Once you have learnt some simple breathing techniques you will have a portable and powerful tool that will help you feel relaxed and in control. You will even sleep better at night.

I advocate 'Active Mindfulness' which is far easier to implement than traditional mindfulness. Most of my clients find it really difficult and let's face it, excruciatingly boring to allocate time to sit and do nothing, even for 10 minutes a day. I advise my clients to practise mindfulness while they are actively on the go. When you are out for a walk, spend a couple of minutes initially. Focus on a few breathes. Then focus on the soles of your feet touching the ground. Then focus on your surrounding environment. You will be amazed how energised you will feel after just a few minutes of 'Active Mindfulness.'

Issues related to ADHD such as impulsivity and self-regulation respond well to mindfulness, as do many aspects of executive function. Spending time in nature can be a form of mindfulness and has been proven to help with focus.

INTENSE EXERCISE

If you want to be able to think with more clarity, or focus on a difficult task, start an intense exercise routine (Berwid, et al. 2012).

Exercise plays a vital role in ADHD management. Health experts recommend five 30-minute exercise sessions per week to manage ADHD symptoms such as mood imbalances, focus and positivity. I have seen with myself and my client how intense exercise really helps the ADHD brain focus, and helps manage the ADHD trait of impulsivity or restlessness.

I advise my clients to do half an hour of intense exercise prior to tackling a boring or complicated task. Even a brisk ten-minute walk works well. As long as you are sweating and your heart is pumping, you should see clear results as your brain wakes up, ready to focus.

Adrian was diagnosed with ADHD. He also suffered from high anxiety, and had made an appointment with his GP to see if he could get some medication. At our first coaching session, I explained to Adrian how exercise was a long-term tool in managing anxiety and depression, and that if done correctly could possibly help him avoid taking medication or at least lessen the dose. Adrian was intrigued. I explained to him that slow and steady was preferable to quick and intense. Over the next few weeks Adrian tried a number of different types of exercises.

He took to cycling with some friends on weekends and joined the local gym. At first he only attended twice a week for half an hour. After a few months he increased the sessions to four times a week, still for 30 minutes. Slowly and steadily, little by little he started to notice a shift in his mood.

He felt more positive and upbeat and much calmer. The inner demon that had previously tormented him was more controllable. Adrian noticed that after an exercise session he could focus better on his work. He now truly understood how critical his exercise routine was in helping him maintain his focus and his positive frame of mind.

Dr. Raun Melmed runs the Melmed Centre in the USA. He specialises in ADHD and ASD. Dr. Melmed issued a very strong statement that if doctors are prescribing ADHD medications without also prescribing other supports such as coaching, they are using the medications off-label, and illegally, because the pharmaceutical companies now clearly state that the medications alone are not enough. He sees the clinics of the future including not just diagnosticians, but care-coordinators, professional organisers, and ADHD coaches. (ACO Conference 2014).

PART 9
CAN I CHANGE
MY HABITS?

CREATE POSITIVE HABITS

Congratulations! You have almost finished this book. If you are like me, and start reading books from the end backwards, then welcome! It doesn't matter where you are along your self-discovery journey. It matters that you are moving forward, little by little. Moving forward means identifying the habits that sabotage your success, and replacing them with new habits. That's all.

There are three parts to every habit:

1. Trigger
2. Routine
3. Gratification

Habits are behaviours that you have done for such a long time that they become subconscious. You don't even think about them. Taking on new habits is a long-term challenge, and covers all areas of life (Wood, et al. 2017). It can take around 3-4 months for the first stage of a habit to be formed. It takes between 3 till 5 years to permanently form a new habit. This is when your brain has formed a permanent pathway. That is a long time; so take a deep breath!

The brain consists of billions of neurons. Each neuron has tens of thousands of branches called dendrites, emerging from its core. The dendrites receive electrical impulses from other neurons and transmit them along a long fibre called the axon. When you commit to a new behaviour, you create new neural networks in the brain. The more you work on a behaviour, the more dendrites are formed, creating new and enriched pathways in your brain.

Recent studies of people in various occupations show that those who carry out more complex work develop more dendrites, leading to enriched neural networks in certain parts of the brain. It can take as little as several weeks or as long as

5 years for new neurons and dendrites to form. This explains why a very high percentage of people who succeeded in weight loss are back to their original weight within 5 years. The new neurons and increased dendrites created in their brains weren't given quite enough time to stabilise before the old habits were reintroduced.

This means that each time you practise a new habit you are strengthening your brain's pathways, making that habit stronger and better established. If you feel stuck it may be that you just need some encouragement and support along the way.

Everyone's life runs on habits – some you're aware of and many that you are not. Taking on board new behaviours and turning them into long-lasting habits takes time. There's no magical solution.

The first step you need to do in dealing with habits is become self-aware. Gather information to understand the cravings that fuel your bad habits and then working out how to change them. A habit could be: smoking, eating too much chocolate, exercising, drinking water, poor family communication, meditating, arriving late/on time to work, handing in reports on time...the list is endless.

You know if you've ever attempted to stop a bad habit that is enjoyable how difficult this is to do. It is also terribly easy to fall back into old habits. This is because the action associated with the bad habit stimulates the brain's pleasure centre. In other words, the nucleus accumbens (a region located near the centre of your brain) releases dopamine, a pleasure hormone into the brain. This explains why your negative habits that may be pleasurable are so difficult to stop.

There are thousands of ways to stop a bad habit and replace it with a new one. However, only one solution will work for you in your unique situation. How do you find it? Do you see what you're up against?

HOW DO YOU CHANGE A HABIT?

There are four points to every habit change:

1. Trigger
2. Routine
3. Gratification
4. Change

You first need to feel uncomfortable enough to want to change the bad habit that isn't serving you well. Next, you should identify the internal or external event that triggers your habit (trigger). The next step is deciding to do something about it. In other words, changing your routine. You will need to increase your self-awareness. Become a scientist for a while. Start to observe your actions around this habit. Don't try changing your behaviour just yet. Just observe. What needs are your gratifying through this habit? You're gathering hard facts. Write down your observations and feelings before during and after you carry out this habit. This may take a few weeks.

The next stage takes time. Once you have identified the gratification you are seeking, focus on adding in an alternative positive routine that you would like to stick with, and go for it, (change). For the next few weeks experiment with different activities that compensate for your current routine, but still give you the gratification you are seeking.

It will take you time to turn the new good behaviour into a habit. On many occasions you may fall back into your old ways. Just try again the next day. Keep up your resolve, and you will start to see slow but steady changes. It's all about deciding where you will channel your efforts and your energy. It is the successful people make the most mistakes! They are willing to take risks and emerge from their comfort zone, try out new experiences and try and try (and try!) again.

Take an idea from this book that has resonated with you,

and put it into action little by little in your life. Don't give up when you slip back into your old habits. Get up and continue moving forward along your journey. You only have one life. Live it well.

If you have more questions now than before you started, then my goal has been achieved! Now go back through this book a second time. Make notes of the various topics you want to look into in more depth. Enjoy your journey of self-discovery.

EPILOGUE

The following idea is attributed to Thomas Armstrong, Phd. Tomorrow morning we will wake up to a culture transformed into flowers. Psychiatrists are now roses. When the sunflower talks to the psychiatrist rose, he gets diagnosed as 'Hugism'. The tiny violet is diagnosed with 'Petal Deficit Disorder'. The Daisy is diagnosed with 'Plainism'. The Orchid is diagnosed with 'Difficultism'. The Rose Psychiatrist sees himself as standard, yet there is no one brain-set that is normal.

Every brain is uniquely wired. We are all neuro-diverse running along a spectrum. No brain is broken. It's a brain that is different. Just as we need bio-diversity on our planet, we need neurodiversity in order to thrive as a society. The Daisy thrives in any soil. The Orchid won't do well in the same soil. Which flowers do we value the most, the Daisy or the Orchid? The Orchid is more trouble to grow, and treasured more because of the difficulty and challenges in growing the flower.

We need to find the right soil for each flower. When we do so, it will thrive and do magnificently. We can't expect the Daisy and the Orchid to thrive in the same soil and do equally well. They need unique environments in which to thrive. No one is broken, they are just neuro-diverse. ADHD brains have strengths and can thrive in environments that appreciate their strengths.

Find the right environment that will support you forward.

STRENGTHS CHART

The purpose of this form is to become more aware of the strengths that you have. Please rank the following strengths in terms of how they impact your life (think about school, work, home, daily functions and social life). After finishing the list, please list your top five strengths in the spaces provided.

Include examples in your life where these top five strengths have been clearly manifest. It may be helpful to make copies of the top 5 strengths and hang them around your home and office, so that as the situations show up you can record as many of the details as you remember.

The more time you spend on this chart, the more self-awareness you will create. Self-awareness is the key to change.

STRENGTH	LOW IMPACT	MEDIUM IMPACT	HIGH IMPACT
1) You come up with new inventions/insights.			
2) You remember easily the jobs you need to do.			
3) When problems crop up you can easily flexibilise yourself to find a solution.			
4) Your sense of humour gets you through life.			

STRENGTH	LOW IMPACT	MEDIUM IMPACT	HIGH IMPACT
5) You are deeply intuitive, understanding things without necessarily knowing why.			
6) You feel in harmony and balanced with nature.			
7) When the going gets tough, if the situation is interesting and in line with your values you will persist to the end.			
8) You are a truth seeker, you find it difficult to be with people who do not have this strength.			
9) You have the courage to do things you believe are the right thing to do.			
10) You are a pioneer.			
11) You are persistent and single minded to reach your goal.			

STRENGTH	LOW IMPACT	MEDIUM IMPACT	HIGH IMPACT
12) You trust your intuition and take risks.			
13) In challenging situations your brain comes alive and you thrive.			
14) You are perceptive to the nuances underlying what people say, and you are usually right.			
15) You have dynamic energy.			
16) You enjoy social situations, you come alive when you are with people.			
17) You are driven to reach my goals. Nothing can stop you, and you get one track minded.			
18) You have the courage to reach out to fulfill your goals.			
19) You constantly have thoughts and ideas coming into your brain.			

STRENGTH	LOW IMPACT	MEDIUM IMPACT	HIGH IMPACT
20) You get easily bored and seek excitement.			
21) When you do something that is in line with your values, you do it perfectly.			
22) You see the perspective of other people.			
23) You learn easily from your mistakes.			
24) In your areas of highest values, you are very organised.			
25) When you are doing work that you love, you hyperfocus, and you are in a flow with time.			
26) You see the big picture.			
27) You see the many details that make up the big picture.			
28) In an emergency you come alive.			

STRENGTH	LOW IMPACT	MEDIUM IMPACT	HIGH IMPACT
29) You have a sense of wonder and fascination in the world around you.			
30) You want to find out the process of how things are done/made.			
31) When a decision is in line with your values, you react impulsively without thinking, and you are usually right.			
32) You have a wisdom beyond your years.			
33) You look and act younger than your years.			
34) You feel balanced and harmonious when you are in nature.			
35) Your thoughts easily entertain you.			
36) You are quick and deep.			
37) People say you are authentic, you are who you are.			

OWN YOUR ADHD

STRENGTH	LOW IMPACT	MEDIUM IMPACT	HIGH IMPACT
38) You have a colourful imagination.			
39) You are a role model to others.			
40) You are deeply committed to causes that you believe in.			

PLEASE FILL IN YOUR TOP 5 STRENGTHS

STRENGTH	1	2	3

(Impact 1,2 or 3)   (Situation)   (Details)

CHALLENGES FORM

Please rate the following challenges in terms of how they impact your life (think about school, work, home, daily functions, social life). After finishing the list, please list your top five challenges in the spaces provided. Include examples in your life where these top five challenges are the most evident.

It is helpful to make copies of the top 5 challenges, and put it in places where you tend to think and write so that as the situations show up you can record as many of the details as you remember. The purpose of this exercise is not to get you depressed! It is to create self-awareness, which is the key to your change. Your challenges are all hidden strengths. You just need to learn some simple tools and understand how you can use them in the right context. They will then move you forward towards your goals.

The more time you spend on this chart, the more self-awareness you will create. Self-awareness is the key to change.

CHALLENGE	LOW IMPACT	MEDIUM IMPACT	HIGH IMPACT
1) Procrastination; you can't get started.			
2) Rumination (thoughts that keep repeating themselves over and over in your mind).			

CHALLENGE	LOW IMPACT	MEDIUM IMPACT	HIGH IMPACT
3) You have a tendency towards perfectionism; constant revising and restarting task or project or being unable to make a decision due to a fear of failure.			
4) Transitioning from thoughts, tasks and situations or from stages in your life is difficult (example, changing schools or jobs or moving or moving from doing a chore to doing homework).			
5) You have energy volatility, from high enthusiasm and energy to being lethargic and tired.			
6) Over promising and not delivering.			
7) When are doing something that you enjoy it is very hard for others or something else to get your attention.			

CHALLENGE	LOW IMPACT	MEDIUM IMPACT	HIGH IMPACT
8) You often blame others for things that aren't right or go wrong in your life.			
9) You have a tendency towards pessimism; thinking you have no talents or strengths.			
10) You have difficulty maintaining relationships for long periods of time.			
11) You say inappropriate things.			
12) You have difficulty paying attention in social, personal, school or work situations.			
13) You have difficulty reading important documents.			

CHALLENGE	LOW IMPACT	MEDIUM IMPACT	HIGH IMPACT
14) You suffer from mood volatility; mood changes suddenly or often throughout the day, you overreact to situations.			
15) You have difficulty reading anything.			
16) You are overly sensitive to other people's comments or opinions of you.			
17) You misread people's remarks or facial expressions.			
18) You have difficulty turning off your brain at night.			
19) You constantly have thoughts and ideas coming into your brain.			
20) You have difficulty sitting still in many situations.			

CHALLENGE	LOW IMPACT	MEDIUM IMPACT	HIGH IMPACT
21) You have difficulty remembering immediate tasks, or going back to tasks if interrupted.			
22) You are frequently late for appointments, school, work, paying bills etc.			
23) You have difficulty making decisions.			
24) You are very disorganised.			
25) You have a hard time sustaining attention.			
26) You have difficulty paying attention to details, you might be able to focus on the big picture but not the pieces that make up the big picture.			

CHALLENGE	LOW IMPACT	MEDIUM IMPACT	HIGH IMPACT
27) You lose or forget things often, especially keys, supplies, homework, important papers, sunglasses etc.			
28) You are easily distracted or lose your train of thought.			
29) You forget to do things, miss appointments, scheduled time with friends, assignment deadlines.			
30) You have difficulties with short-term memory.			
31) You react impulsively or impatiently (shout out answers, don't wait for your turn, impulse spending, race through tests and don't check answers).			

CHALLENGE	LOW IMPACT	MEDIUM IMPACT	HIGH IMPACT
32) You suffer from poor planning and time-management skills, you often feel like you have been working for a long periods of time, but you are not getting anything done.			
33) You make careless errors.			
34) You have trouble with multiple step operation, you can't sustain attention, forget steps.			
35) You often feel overwhelmed, and your brain may feel paralysed, and you may feel anxious.			
36) Your physical environment is often a mess and disorganised.			

CHALLENGE	LOW IMPACT	MEDIUM IMPACT	HIGH IMPACT
37) When making decisions you often don't think things through and/or consider the ramifications.			
38) You wait until the last minute to get things done, due to poor planning or time management problems, or your brain needs extra stimulation and adrenaline to get things done.			
39) You appear thoughtless or unconcerned, you may be thinking about something else or not recognise the reality of what someone is trying to convey to you.			
40) You have difficulty giving yourself credit for your achievements or recognising your strengths.			

PLEASE FILL IN YOUR TOP 5 CHALLENGES

CHALLENGE	1	2	3

(Impact 1,2 or 3) (Situation)   (Details)

ADHD SELF-TEST

This test will give you a sense of whether or not you may have ADHD/ADD. It is not a diagnostic tool, and will not replace a full assessment by a psychiatrist or qualified ADHD nurse.

Answer "yes" "no" to the following answers.

There are 18 quick questions: The first 9 explore inattention and focus.

The symptoms need to be visible in multiple settings, such as work, home, college and have been present since a young age or teen years.

PLEASE NOTE: ADHD/ADD is a spectrum condition. There are a range of symptoms and severity. Some symptoms may be a constant challenge for you, others rarely if ever. The symptoms in girls and women may differ to the symptoms in boys and men. Women may suffer more from anxiety and depression. This means that the core ADHD symptoms are often masked.

PART 1 - INATTENTION

POOR ATTENTION TO DETAIL – I often make careless mistakes in school work and other activities. I skim read. I get small details wrong and make simple errors because I fail to pay attention.

POOR LISTENER – During long conversations I tune out the speaker. I often miss parts of the conversation because my mind has wandered off. Sometimes I lose my train of thought and wander off on a tangent.

INTERNALLY DISTRACTED – I struggle to remain focused during lectures, lengthy reading and conversations. I find it difficult to finish long and complex tasks, even leisure activities. I often do a few tasks at once. I get distracted by my inner world. I am often lost in thought imagining ideas and scenarios. I am clever but a bit absent minded.

EXTERNALLY DISTRACTED – I get distracted by my external environment. I find it difficult to filter out the outside stimuli.

I AM FORGETFUL – I forget appointments, and buy duplicates of items that I forgot I owned.

DIFFICULTY FOLLOWING INSTRUCTIONS – I dislike following instructions. I like to do things my own way. I struggle to keep to routines and schedules. I know what I should do, I just don't do it.

DISORGANISED – I have problems with organisation. I have paper piles everywhere. I procrastinate and get overwhelmed. I have problems with organising my finances and my thoughts.

AVOIDING TASKS THAT NEED SUSTAINED MENTAL EFFORT – I do not like to engage in tasks that require sustained mental effort and focus.

I MISPLACE THINGS WAY TOO OFTEN – I often lose important documents, keys phone etc. I seem to put things down and then I can't find them again. I have piles of paper and clutter around my space.

The threshold score for PART 1 is at least 5 "yes" answers. If you score less than 5 it suggests it may be something else.

You may be overly stressed by a stressful situation such as a recent divorce, a death in the family, job loss, or other life change. It might also be any one of a number of medical issues. It may be helpful to talk this over with your GP.

If you scored 5 and above then you may have ADD, the Predominantly Inattentive Subtype of ADHD. You may struggle with attention and distractibility. You may be forgetful, sensitive to your environment, easily distracted, or overwhelmed by busy situations.

Many adults with undiagnosed ADHD find coping strategies, (not always healthy ones) to cope with their challenges. Around 50% of children who have been diagnosed with ADHD as children grow out of their symptoms, but around 50% still do suffer from them for life, and need ADHD meds and life skills to help them access their potential. If you still feel focus, overwhelm, and distraction are a problem consider what your answers would have been back in primary school would your score have been higher?

Learn more about ADHD, and see what resonates with you. The coping tools that adults with ADHD use to manage their ADHD can help anyone who is overwhelmed and stressed.

PART 2 – IMPULSIVITY AND HYPERACTIVITY

The next 6 questions focus on your hyperactivity, and the last 3 questions focus on your impulsivity. You probably don't bounce off the walls like a hyperactive child, but perhaps you often feel restless and driven, like there's an engine inside you.

Maybe your thoughts are racing, sometimes tumbling, ricocheting as you pour out one idea after another.

You may crave excitement and trying new things. Or love highly stimulating activities with a big pay-off.

Read the following questions, answer, "yes" or "no" and find out if you have an element of hyperactivity and impulsivity.

NON-STOP TALKING – I talk a lot. I tell great stories, and don't have patience to hear others out. If someone else tries to speak, I may get louder if I feel pressured to say my piece.

PHYSICAL RESTLESSNESS – I often feel restless during long meetings/classes. I find it very difficult to sit still, and need to fidget to focus.

DIFFICULTY RELAXING – I find it difficult to unwind and relax. Making conversation for its own sake is so boring. I often rush into and past things because I haven't got the patience to work it through.

MENTAL RESTLESSNESS – My mind is always moving, and making new connections. I have had many different jobs and have moved around a lot.

I AM INTERNALLY DRIVEN – I have an engine that is always pushing me forward, I can't seem to sit still for a minute. I move on and on, until I crash. I can hyperfocus on hobbies that excite me, and then when I get bored, I simply move on. I sprint rather than run a marathon.

I NEED TO MOVE – I wish I could have "walking meetings" Doing nothing hurts my brain and gets me upset.

INTERRUPTING – I don't have patience to wait for others to finish speaking, and often interrupt before the person has finished speaking. I often dominate conversations because I get excited.

WAITING IS TORTURE – I hate long queues and slow traffic is maddeningly frustrating. I hate waiting for other people. Spare me the details, just give over the bare points.

BLURTING – My mind races and I have to get out what I say right now. I don't have patience to hear people out and I interrupt them before they have finished what they say. I say "yes" to things without thinking things through. Then I am left with too many commitments, and I feel totally overwhelmed.

If you have scored under 5 out of 9, you may have the Combined Subtype of ADHD.

While most people struggle with some of these symptoms, that doesn't mean they have ADHD. They could be stressed by major life events or any number of medical issues. But your score suggests a full assessment by a specialist who understands ADHD might be in order

You struggle with Hyperactivity and Impulsivity. You may feel restless, talkative, impatient, and have strong emotions. But also driven, curious, creative, with excess energy, and needing to be on the go. Problems with Attention, Restlessness, and Impulsivity make up the Combined Subtype of ADHD. This is the most common form of ADHD.

If you have the combined type of ADHD you struggle with attention and distractibility. You may be forgetful, sensitive, distracted, or overwhelmed by hectic situations. You may be poor at listening, your thoughts wander, you tune out. As well, you may be hyper-sensitive to loud noise, busy places, a light touch, or strong odours.

With all types of ADHD you may be overwhelmed when watching scary videos, or stressful situations. You may lose track of what you and others are saying, what you were meant to be doing, or forget people's names.

While most people struggle with some of these symptoms, that doesn't mean they have ADHD. You could be stressed by major life events or any number of medical issues. But a score above 5 suggests that a full assessment by an ADHD psychiatrist might be in order.

ABOUT THE AUTHOR

Faigy is a mum of 5 children, with more than one ADHD child. Faigy is a Pioneer, Trailblazer, and a Visionary Disrupter. She is a staunch advocate for ADHD women. Faigy is the first ADHD coach to achieve PAAC certification on the PCAC level in the UK. This is the Gold Standard for ADHD Coaching credentialing, worldwide.

Faigy is passionate about ADHD education and empowerment. Having ADHD herself, and being an ADHD mum, she has a unique understanding of the challenges and strengths of ADHD, she is proof that you can live your successful life with your ADHD.

Faigy coaches adults, students and parents for their ADHD children.

In 2019 Faigy founded the Creative Women in Business Mastermind group, the first of its kind in the UK.

https://focuswithfaigy.com/business-networking-for-adhd-women/

She is part of the APPG for ADHD, a lobbying group that meets quarterly in the House of Commons. The APPG advocates for improved assessment and treatment for children and adults with ADHD in the UK.

Faigy is on the coaching committee for ADHD Europe.

She appears regularly on the Men's and Women's Radio Stations, which promote mental health awareness.

https://soundcloud.com/womensradiostation/know-your-therapy-with-bernadette-bruckner-faigy-liebermann-adhd-coach

Faigy mentors ADHD coaches how to come out of their own way and establish their dream ADHD coaching business with ease.

Join the Facebook group for ADHD coaches. Benefit from FREE training and resources.

www.facebook.com/groups/448409712721774/

Website: www.focuswithfaigy.com

ABOUT ORGANISE PRO

Faigy has been a Professional Organiser since 2013. Faigy has been training Professional Organisers since 2015. Organise Pro offers bespoke Professional Organiser Training together with a foolproof business model. Organise Pro offers additional training upgrades on topics related to Professional Organising throughout the year.

All Programs focus on the ADHD aspect of clutter and disorganisation, and are tailored for clients and Professional Organisers who are creative ADHD women.

The Program emphasises "Organised and systemised, NOT neat and tidy." Join the Facebook group for professional organisers. Members get access to FREE training and resources.

www.facebook.com/groups/theorganiseproinnercircle/
Website: www.organisepro.com

ABOUT 'BANISH YOUR OVERWHELM - DECLUTTER YOUR LIFE'

A decluttering guide for women with ADHD.

This is Part 1 in a two-part series on home organisation for women with ADHD or ADHD tendencies.

When you want to organise your home, you first need to declutter. When this stage has been successfully completed, you can then organise what you have left.

In this book you will learn about the underlying neuroscience that may be making it difficult for you to part with your clutter. The book is full of hands-on practical tools how to bravely face your clutter, and part with it once and for all, thereby banishing or greatly diminishing your feelings of overwhelm and your anxiety.

Discover how to liberate yourself from your anxiety and overwhelm. Open the door to your focus and clarity.

You *can* live your successful life with your ADHD.

Book available in hardcopy and kindle format.

Buy online at www.focuswithfaigy.com

ABOUT 'BANISH YOUR OVERWHELM - SIMPLIFY YOUR LIFE'

This book is the second book in the 'Banish Your Overwhelm' series. This book is tailored for ADHD women, or for women who have ADHD tendencies.

You will learn how to support your ADHD and create your Simplified Life. As a wife, mum and businesswoman living successfully with ADHD, I am proof that you can do it.

Have you ever wondered what goes on during a Professional Organiser session? Discover what it is like to work with a Professional Organiser. Meet Sandra, and follow her journey from cluttered, and overwhelmed to organised and focused. Lots of stories and photos throughout the book.

My clients call me "Fairy" since, after an organising session, it seems like I have waved a magic wand to banish their clutter to oblivion and simplify their lives. Sorry to disappoint you, I don't yet possess a magic wand. I do possess my magic formula for your ADHD success "Simplify, Systemise, Success." With the right tools that are focused for your ADHD brain, you *can* create your Simplified ADHD Life.

Book available in hardcopy and kindle format.

Buy online at www.focuswithfaigy.com

FURTHER READING

- Faigy Liebermann, *'Banish Your Overwhelm – Declutter Your Life'*
- Faigy Liebermann, *'Banish Your Overwhelm – Simplify Your Life'*
- Lindsey Biel and Nancy Peske, *'Raising a Sensory Smart Child'*
- Peg Dawson and Richard Guare, *'Smart but Scattered'*
- Dr. Lara Honos-Webb, *'The Gift of Adult ADD'*
- Ross Greene, *'The Explosive Child'*
- Dr. Edward Hallowell, *'Driven to Distraction'*
- Sari Solden, *'Women with Attention Deficit Disorder'*
- Lydia Zylowski, *'The Mindfulness Prescription for ADHD'*

REFERENCES

AADD-UK (2018). Comorbidities. Retrieved from https://aadduk.org/symptoms-diagnosis-treatment/comorbidities/. Accessed 17/1/19.

Additude Editors (2018). ADHD by the numbers. Retrieved from https://www.additudemag.com/the-statistics-of-adhd/. Accessed 1/7/18.

Additude Editors (2018). The glorious comeback of the gap year (thank you, Malia Obama). Retrieved from https://www.additudemag.com/slideshows/the-glorious-comeback-of-the-gap-year-thank-you-malia-obama/. Accessed 1/7/18.

ADHD statistics in the UK. Retrieved from https://www.bbc.co.uk/news/uk-england-44956540. Accessed 1/12/18.

Altszuler, A. R., Page, T. F., Gnagy, E. et al. (2016). Financial Dependence of Young Adults with Childhood ADHD. Journal of Abnormal Child Psychology, 44(6), 1217-29. DOI: 10.1007/s10802-015-0093-9. Accessed 12/12/18.

Barkley, R. A. (2010). Taking Charge of ADHD, Third Edition: The Complete, Authoritative Guide for Parents. New York, New York: The Guilford Press. Accessed 2/7/18.

Berwid, O. G., & Halperin, J. M. (2012). Emerging Support for a Role of Exercise in Attention-Deficit/Hyperactivity Disorder Intervention Planning. Current Psychiatry Reports, 14(5), 543-51. DOI: 10.1007/s11920-012-0297-4. Accessed 1/12/18.

Cherkasova, M., Sulla, E. M., Dalena, K. L. et al. (2013). Developmental Course of Attention Deficit Hyperactivity Disorder and its Predictors. Journal of the Canadian Academy of Child and Adolescent Psychiatry, 22(1), 47-54. https://www.ncbi.nlm.nih.gov/pmc/articles/PMC3565715/. Accessed 12/12/18.

Chupetlovska-Anastasova, A. (2014). Longitudinal

exploration of friendship patterns of children and early adolescents with and without Attention-Deficit/Hyperactivity Disorder (Doctoral Dissertation). Retrieved from http://citeseerx.ist.psu.edu. Accessed 1/11/18.

Cortese, S., Konofal, E., Lecendreux, M. (2008). The Relationship Between Attention-Deficit-Hyperactivity-Disorder and Restless Leg Syndrome. European Neurological Review, 3(1), 111-114. DOI:http://doi.org/10.17925/ENR.2008.03.01.111. Accessed 1/11/18.

Dawson, P., Guare, R. (2018). Executive Skills in Children and Adolescents, Third Edition: A Practical Guide to Assessment and Intervention. New York, NY: The Guilford Press. Accessed 12/12/18.

Demontis, D., Walters, R. K., Martin, J. et al. (2017). 'Discovery of the first genome-wide significant risk loci for attention deficit/hyperactivity disorder. Nature Genetics (2018). Available at https://www.nature.com/articles/s41588-018-0269-7. Accessed 12/12/18.

DrSusanYoung (2018) 18 October. Congrats @ErynnBrook on this concise summary of #ADHD. Greatest comorbidity is conduct disorder in childhood. 30% of youth and 26% of adult offenders in prison have ADHD. Most (80%) are undiagnosed. Females, generally, are totally under the radar [Tweet]. Retrieved from https://twitter.com/DrSusanYoung1. Accessed 19/10/18.

Faraone, S. V., Sergeant, J., Gillberg, C. et al. (2003). The worldwide prevalence of ADHD: is it an American condition? World psychiatry: Official Journal of the World Psychiatric Association (WPA), 2(2), 104-13. https://www.ncbi.nlm.nih.gov/pmc/articles/PMC1525089/. Accessed 31/12/18.

Fernandez, E., Bergado Rosado, J. A., Rodriguez Perez, D. et al. (2018). 'Effectiveness of a computer-based training program of attention and memory in patients with acquired brain damage', Behav. Sci. 2018;8(1), 4; doi:10.3390/bs8010004. Accessed 2/1/19.

Ferrin, M., Perez-Ayala, V., El-Abd, S. et al. (2016). A randomised controlled trial evaluating the efficacy of a psychoeducation program for families of children and adolescents with ADHD in the UK: results after a 6-month follow-up. Journal of Attention Disorders. Accessed 2/1/19.

Field, S., Parker, D., Sawilowsky, S. et al. (2010, August 31). Quantifying the Effectiveness of Coaching for College Students with Attention Deficit/Hyperactivity Disorder: Final Report to the Edge Foundation. Retrieved from https://edgefoundation.org/wp-content/uploads/2016/07/Wayne-State-Research-Executive-Summary.pdf. Accessed 8/1/19.

Fuermaier, A. B. M., Tucha, L., Koerts J. et al. (2013). Complex prospective memory in adults with Attention Deficit Hyperactivity Disorder. PLOS ONE 8(3): e58338. https://doi.org/10.1371/journal.pone.0058338. Accessed 10/1/19.

Green, A. L., Rabiner, D. L. (2012). What Do We Really Know About ADHD in College Students? Neurotherapeutics: The Journal of the American Society for Experimental Neurotherapeutics, 9(3), 559-68. DOI: 10.1007/s13311-012-0127-8. Accessed 10/1/19.

Harpin, V. A. (2005). The effect of ADHD on the life of an individual, their family, and community from preschool to adult life. Archives of Disease in Childhood, 90 Suppl 1:i2-7. DOI: 10.1136/adc.2004.059006. Accessed 6/6/18.

Harris, M. N., Voigt, R. G., Barbaresi, W. J. et al. (2013). ADHD and learning disabilities in former late preterm infants: a population-based birth cohort. Pediatrics, 132(3), e630-6. https://www.ncbi.nlm.nih.gov/pmc/articles/PMC3876753/. Accessed 14/10/18.

Jacobson, R. (2018). How to Help Kids with Working Memory Issues. Retrieved from https://childmind.org/article/how-to-help-kids-with-working-memory-issues/. Accessed 14/11/18.

Jaroslawska, A.J., Gathercole, S.E., Allen, R, J, et al. (2016). Following instructions from working memory: Why does action at encoding and recall help? Memory & Cognition, 44(8), 1183–1191. DOI: 10.3758/s13421-016-0636-5. Accessed 13/11/18.

Kent, K. M., Pelham, W. E., Molina, B. S., et al. (2011). The Academic Experience of Male High School Students with ADHD. Journal of Abnormal Child Psychology, 39(3), 451-62. DOI: 10.1007/s10802-010-9472-4. Accessed 12/12/18.

Knouse, L. E., & Safren, S. A. (2010). Current Status of Cognitive Behavioural Therapy for Adult Attention-Deficit Hyperactivity Disorder. The Psychiatric Clinics of North America, 33(3), 497-509. DOI: 10.1016/j.psc.2010.04.001. Accessed 12/12/18.

Lange, W. K., et al., (2010). The history of attention deficit hyperactivity disorder. Retrieved from US national library of medicine national institutes of health. https://www.ncbi.nlm.nih.gov/pmc/articles/PMC3000907/. Accessed 1/7/18.

Lezak, M. (1979). Recovery of Memory and Learning Functions Following Traumatic Brain Injury. Cortex, 15 (1), 63-72. https://doi.org/10.1016/S0010-9452(79)80007-6. Accessed 1/7/18.

Loe, I.M., Feldman, H.M., (2007). Academic and Educational Outcomes of Children With ADHD. Pediatric Psychology, 32(6), 643-654. https://doi.org/10.1093/jpepsy/jsl054. Accessed 2/12/18.

Matthies, S, Philipsen, A. (2016). Comorbidity of Personality Disorders and Adult Attention Deficit Hyperactivity Disorder (ADHD)--Review of Recent Findings. Current Psychiatry Reports, 18(33). https://doi.org/10.1007/s11920-016-0675-4. Accessed 12/12/18.

McEwen, B.S. (2007). Physiology and Neurobiology of Stress and Adaptation: central role of the brain. Physiological Reviews, 87(3), 873-904. https://doi.org/10.1152/physrev.00041.2006. Accessed 10/11/18.

Mesman, J., Van Ijzendoorn, M.H., et al. (2009). The Many Faces of the Still-Face Paradigm: A Review and Meta-Analysis. Developmental Review, 29(2), 120-162. https://doi.org/10.1016/j.dr.2009.02.001. Retrieved 11/11/18.

Mitchell, J.T., Zylowska, L., Kollins, S.H. (2015). Mindfulness Meditation Training for Attention-Deficit/Hyperactivity Disorder in Adulthood: Current Empirical Support, Treatment Overview, and Future Directions. Cognitive and Behavioral Practice, 22(2), 172-191. DOI: 10.1016/j.cbpra.2014.10.002. Accessed 2/7/18.

Polanczyk, G., de Lima, M.S., Horta, B.L. et al. (2007). The Worldwide Prevalence of ADHD: A Systematic Review and Metaregression Analysis. The American Journal of Psychiatry, 164(6):942-8. Accessed 10/10/18. https://ajp.psychiatryonline.org/doi/abs/10.1176/ajp.2007.164.6.942?url_ver=Z39.88-2003&rfr_id=ori:rid:crossref.org&rfr_dat=cr_pub%3dpubmed. Accessed 10/10/18.

Prevatt, F., Yelland, S. (2015). An Empirical Evaluation of ADHD Coaching in College Students. Journal of Attention Disorders, 19(8), 666-77. DOI: 10.1177/1087054713480036. Accessed 10/10/18.

Ptacek, R., Stefano, G. B., Weissenberger, S., et al. (2016). Attention Deficit Hyperactivity Disorder and Disordered Eating Behaviors: Links, Risks, and Challenges Faced. Neuropsychiatric Disease and Treatment, 12, 571-9. DOI:10.2147/NDT.S68763. Accessed 11/12/18.

Quinn, P. O., & Madhoo, M. (2014). A Review of Attention-Deficit/Hyperactivity Disorder in Women and Girls: Uncovering This Hidden Diagnosis. The Primary Care Companion for CNS Disorders, 16(3), PCC.13r01596.

Accessed 1/2/19.

Robinson, J. (2013). Three-Quarters of Your Doctor Bills are Because of This. Retrieved from https://www.huffingtonpost.com/joe-robinson/stress-and-health_b_3313606.html. Accessed 1/2/19

Singh, A, Yeh C.J., Verma, N. et al. (2015). Overview of Attention Deficit Hyperactivity Disorder in Young Children. Health Psychology Research, 3(2). DOI: 10.4081/hpr.2015.2115. Accessed 30/1/19.Accessed 17/7/18.

Smith, B.H., Molina, B.S.G., Pelham, W.E. (2002). The Clinically Meaningful Link Between Alcohol Use and Attention Deficit Hyperactivity Disorder. Alcohol Research & Health, 26(2), 122-129.Accessed 7/7/18.

Steiner, N., J., Frenette, E., C., Rene K. M., et al. (2013). In-School Neurofeedback Training for ADHD: Sustained Improvements from a Randomized Control Trial. Pediatrics 133 (March 2014 issue 3). Available at http://pediatrics.aappublications.org/content/133/3/483 doi:1 0.1542/peds.2013-2059. Accessed 6/7/18.

Svedlund, N. E., Norring, C., Ginsberg, Y., et al. (2017). Symptoms of Attention Deficit Hyperactivity Disorder (ADHD) Among Adult Eating Disorder Patients. BMC Psychiatry, 17(1), 19. DOI:10.1186/s12888-016-1093-1. Accessed 1/12/18.

Wilens, T. E., & Spencer, T. J. (2010). Understanding attention-deficit/hyperactivity disorder from childhood to adulthood. Postgraduate medicine, 122(5), 97-109. DOI: 10.3810/pgm.2010.09.2206. Accessed 3/10/18.

Wood, W., Neal, D.T., (2016). Healthy Through Habit: Interventions for Initiating and Maintaining Health Behavior Change. Behavioral Science & Policy, 2(1), 70-83. https://behavioralpolicy.org/wp-content/uploads/2017/05/BSP_vol1is1_Wood.pdf. Accessed 3/9/18.

Zametkin, A.J., Nordahl, T.E., et al. (1990). Cerebral Glucose Metabolism in Adults with Hyperactivity of

OWN YOUR ADHD

Childhood Onset. The New England Journal of Medicine, 323(20):1361-6. DOI:10.1056/NEJM199011153232001 https://www.researchgate.net/scientific-contributions/39786703_Alan_J_Zametkin. Accessed 12/1/18.

Printed in Great Britain
by Amazon